IN THE BLINK OF AN EYE

*The Story of Mia Austin and Her Triumph
Over Locked-In Syndrome*

MIA L AUSTIN
WITH SUE KELSO RYAN

To order additional copies of this book, contact:
Xlibris
1-888-795-4274
www.Xlibris.com
Orders@Xlibris.com

They say live life to the full,
but no one listens.
They should.

INTRODUCTION

—⁓∿⟋⊙⟍⊙⟋⊙⟍⊙⟋⟍∿—

The Big Bang

I must have woken on the morning of the 16th November 2009 totally oblivious as to what was going to happen because I'd been to work as usual, nothing different, followed by the gym where I did my normal workout. I got home and went for a bath and then BAM!

Welcome to my story all about me. Now you can get into the head of a stroke victim.

So, here's the key...

CHAPTER 1

About Me

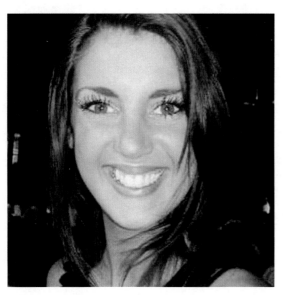

Let me introduce myself… my name is Mia Austin. I was twenty-one when my life was turned around by a massive stroke, leaving me unable to talk, move or eat. I will paint a brief picture of my life before I tell you my story. I am the girl next door; the feisty one. At the time, I had everything going for me: an amazing family and incredible friends and I also had a long-term boyfriend, we were even saving for a mortgage together. I didn't drink (or not often) and didn't smoke. I had the best childhood where my parents were both teachers, so I had a great educational background. I had been in my dream job, working at a travel agency, since I was 16. Here I met some of the best friends; friends that have stuck by me through tough times, and I had just been offered an educational trip with them to Disneyland Florida. Who knew everything could change in one night?

So on 'the night', I had been to the gym but had left a bit earlier than usual because I just didn't feel right about myself. I had plans to go out with my mates that night but had to flake on them because I just needed to get home, I felt awful with a banging headache/ migraine and all shaky and faint.

As I pulled up outside my home in my car, I saw my Mum in the front room window pretending to be slaving away ironing. I went straight in to her, telling her how badly I'd done at the gym and she replied, 'There's always tomorrow…'

HOW IRONIC.

Anyway, she didn't need much persuasion for me to finish her ironing while she made my tea for me. After I had finished my tea I still felt extremely rough, so I went up to run a bath thinking maybe that might help; but before I had even finished running it, I had to suddenly lie down and put my head on the cold tiles of the bathroom floor because my head had suddenly become incredibly sore and I was unable to cope with the pain.

A minute or two later as I went to stand up I fainted, banging the back of my head really hard on the bathroom radiator.

Reflecting back on this week of my life, there were perhaps some obvious signs of what was to come; while I was busy packing my bags for a trip of a lifetime, I was still suffering from really bad headaches and nausea. I had been getting really bad headaches for a few months before and no-one took me seriously, including the doctors. Looking back, they were a definitely sign of what was about to happen.

999

I managed to get myself down the stairs to my Mum and Dad and I told them how I felt and that I had fainted. Dad said, 'Go to bed, babe.' So, as you do when you're ill, I went to sleep in their bed, I was later sick and worryingly grey. My Dad, thank god, knew I wasn't right and rang 999.

I was terrified and couldn't walk or think straight, so the ambulance guys stretchered me downstairs and out to the ambulance. Mum came in with me and Dad, followed in the car.

Thank goodness for Dad's instinct because in the ambulance I kept losing consciousness and then my left side just went and I lost my voice and all sensation.

PANIC SET IN!!!

Hospital One

The ambulance took me to Hospital One, a short drive from my home on the Wirral. When I arrived at the hospital I was so frightened but the nurses were just chatting intently and it didn't seem as though I was important in the slightest. Next thing I know, I'm drifting in and out of consciousness.

Initially, I thought I was having an out of body experience as I could clearly see my friends, family and doctors surrounding me. I tried to ask my family what had happened but they didn't respond. I soon acknowledged that they couldn't hear me, as I was Mumbling. Many thoughts crossed my mind in this moment. Had I just come out of throat surgery? Surely not, as I soon realised I couldn't move one bone in my body. At first, I felt as if I was buried alive.

Unfortunately, I wasn't offered any scans or clot busting drugs at first, as they were not sure what was going on and were actually treating me for swine flu at one point. I feel like a lot of time was wasted before the correct diagnosis – a catastrophic stroke – time that could have made all the difference. It was only later on that they did brain scans and checked for clots.

What is a Stroke?

After research I have found out that blood clots are the most frequent causes of strokes. In my case, I had a blood clot, which caused the stroke to occur. So, what is the reason that this happened? The bad thing is no-one has ever told me the reason, so I can't prevent it happening again. Once you've had a stroke, you have a one-in-three chance of having another within three years.

I was fit and healthy; I went to the gym most nights and spent most Sundays mountain climbing (the reason that my charity is called Mountains for Mia). I didn't drink often and had never smoked. I was a travel agent who had high ambitions in the travel industry and I would put myself under a great deal of pressure, trying to make sure that my customers had the perfect holiday. At the time, I was also really stressed about money because my then-boyfriend and I were desperately saving to get on the property ladder.

Stress is a risk factor for having a stroke. Experts believe it's possible that stress may cause inflammation in the body, which can lead to stroke or heart attack. Being stressed over a long period of time means that stress hormones increase your blood pressure, and that's the leading cause of stroke. Stress hormones can cause diseases such as diabetes, atherosclerosis, and heart disease – which all increase your risk of having a stroke. Strokes are caused by a decreased blood supply to the brain, starving it of oxygen. In older adults, the most frequent cause is a blood clot that forms inside the heart or a blood vessel and travels to the brain. I fall into the category of younger stroke patients and research has shown that up to 25 percent of strokes in patients under the age of 45 are caused by clots. The majority of strokes in the younger age group are caused by brain haemorrhages. Some strokes are due to genetic factors, malformation of blood vessels leading to haemorrhage and possibly even the amount of coffee you drink!

First Stop - Intensive Care

Soon after I was admitted and before my family had seen me properly, a team of solemn faced doctors took them into a room for a meeting. Everyone thought that was it and the doctors confirmed that it could be. They broke the news to my family that I wasn't going to make it through the night and to prepare for the worst. My Mum said the family all took the news in different ways and said that her first thought was that she didn't want me to pass away in the hospital; what a thought for a mother to have to think about. The doctors said they could move me to a private room and that I could have all my family in with me and play my music. From this meeting, my Mum walked straight to the room they had put me in, tears streaming down her face, and she started calling my name. Then I woke up in a panic and I opened my eyes: She didn't expect that! It was the first time that I had opened my eyes since being in hospital. She shouted and all the doctors came rushing in.

Fuck

I remember being taken for a lumbar puncture and at that point I was on a life support machine. They decided to put me into an induced coma to help my brain recover, which lasted six days. My family were notified I had had a stroke and would never walk or talk again because I had a blood clot which caused a stroke to follow. They diagnosed me with locked-in syndrome.

I was so confused and agitated (apparently that's very common under the circumstances). When I first woke up in the hospital, I was seriously disorientated. When I first opened my eyes, I was desperately trying to work out my surroundings; I was attached to all these machines with my PJ top cut open. As I was so high on the medical drugs they had given me, it took a long time to figure out where I was. Where was I? Why could no one hear me? Why couldn't I move? What had happened? But I was just too exhausted to investigate.

My family took it in turns to sit with me so I was never on my own. The nurses were so lovely and kind to my family but I was unaware of all that. As I have done my research, I have found out that it is common for people who have had brain injuries and have gone into a coma to have anger outbursts when waking up, however it is not their fault; some people don't have any recollection of what has happened, so they are confused and disorientated.

Apparently, one night while I was in the coma, my Mum, sister Sophie and boyfriend Rich were with me and there was a patient, who thought Sophie was a nurse. He was waiting for his family to arrive from abroad, and he asked my Mum to sing Perry Como, so she did: Magic Moments. Then Sophie sang some songs - it must have been surreal: people clinging onto life with a bit of "Austin time" thrown in. Another patient thought my sister Sophie was Roxy Mitchell from Eastenders and I started hallucinating that everyone was standing at the end of the bed holding huge placards protesting to get me to open my eyes.

What I Remember

My recollection of intensive care was that it was horrendous but the best care, where I was in the best hands. Observations were taken every fifteen minutes. People assume that while you're in a coma you're completely unresponsive, but I remember everything. I remember who was sitting with me each day and them all begging, 'Please, please wake up!' and my extremely strange dreams. I woke from the induced coma to the sound of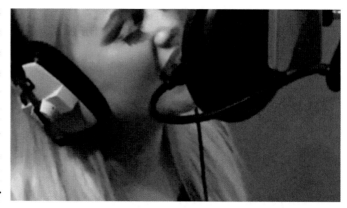
my sister singing and my little Mum in her dungarees. I imagined my sister singing in a concert to me but it turns out that while I was in the coma, they were playing me a CD of her singing the Leonard Cohen song, *Hallelujah*. I was thinking, 'What the hell is going on? What am I doing here?' I remember trying to speak but not being able to.

I had tubes all over my face. Doctors told me that I had suffered an extremely serious stroke which led to being stuck with Locked-in Syndrome. I thought to myself that I ultimately had to make the decision: to fight for the life I wanted to live, or to give up. But, of course, I chose to fight for my health and deal with this tragedy. So this was it; it was now or never, I had to take over breathing for myself. Not once have I ever regretted my decision to go on living my life.

The following week was a blur, or perhaps I have just chosen not to remember it. My sister would sit with one of the old men, who was clearly coming to the end of his life and had no family and she would sing to him. It was a harrowing experience, not for me but watching the people around me.

Once I had comprehended what had happened to me, I needed to answer the many questions my family had. The doctor rapidly taught me to use the only working part of me, which was my eyes. I was taught to communicate through eye movements that seemed so simple, eyes up for 'yes' and eyes down for 'no'. However, this became extremely tiring.

I should emphasise that I had no clue at that time what locked-in syndrome was at all. To me it was just some medical jargon; it meant nothing to me, but I was curious about the stroke because I knew that was a real thing. So I would interrogate everyone, which was really unfair of me but everyone was protecting me by keeping the truth from me. It was a kind thought but I needed answers about why I wasn't in control of my body.

I needed to know things like was my face drooped?
How long would this last?
I thought a stroke meant one side of your body still worked?
Stroke awareness adverts suggest that you have a fire in your brain so was I left with brain damage?

I finally got Rich's attention and opened my eyes widely until he guessed I wanted to know and as he explained it finally all this made sense and I understood what had happened... I just don't understand why this happened... why did this happen to me?
I thought, 'I guess I'll have to ride this one out.'
To think, two months before I was celebrating at my 21st birthday party... This was MADNESS!!!

Before I was able to get answers to all my questions, I was moved on to my next destination. They wanted the bed and the room my family had been staying in.

What is Locked-in Syndrome?

Locked-in Syndrome (LIS) is the result of a traumatic injury to the brain stem, possibly as a result of a stroke, heart attack or brain haemorrhage, and it leaves the patient completely paralysed: unable to speak, eat or move any of their body, other than their eyes. Usually, they are still just as capable intellectually as before the injury – hence the term, 'locked-in'. Involuntary movements, such as breathing, aren't affected and they are often still able to feel sensations, such as pain. Some patients recover some of their mobility but it's rare to get much movement back and almost unheard of to recover completely. There are records of patients whose medical team didn't recognise that they were conscious – sometimes their awareness was only recognised when family members noticed tiny vertical eye movements or blinking. There are also accounts of patients who endured months or years without mental stimulation because they were thought to be unconscious. These days, doctors can use brain scans to show that there is activity and hence awareness but even today it can take months to diagnose LIS.

High Dependency

I was moved to the high dependency ward and everyone around me wanted to keep everything as normal as possible. My sister and Rich would watch the X-Factor and films with me. Everyone had to come in aprons and I remember laughing to myself and thinking, 'Oh god, who dressed him today?'

CHAPTER 2

Introducing; My Family

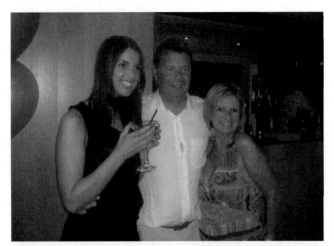

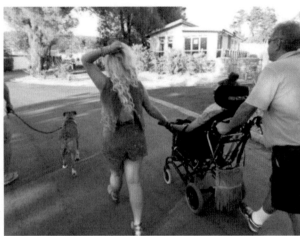

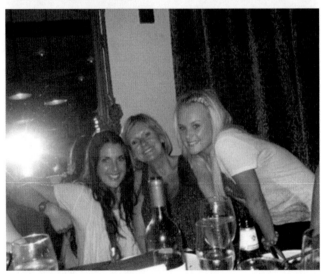

At this point, I should probably introduce my family – my greatest support. There's my Mum and Dad, older brother Sam and younger sister Sophie. You'll be hearing a lot about them, as well as all the wonderful friends and carers who have helped me to get to where I am today.

At the time I had a boyfriend, Rich, and we had been together three years before the stroke. It was true love; I thought this was it he was the one. We were even saving for our mortgage together. When the accident happened, he was there for me every step of the way and he was a big part of the reason I wanted to open my eyes to see him again.

Second Stop

So I was transferred to Ward 2 …

This was a single room at the end of the ward. Such poorly people! Anyway, there I was… but there was no 24-hour care, so my good old Dad created havoc and they provided me with a nurse overnight. I found it very trying, as I couldn't communicate. I was there a week. I had visitors and family, but no-one really had a clue how to help me. One day, before Mum and Sophie arrived, a nurse chopped some of my hair off! When they arrived, Sophie went mental and left a very angry note on my notes to say how she felt about that. It probably included some very strong language.

A patient called Susan thought my room was a smoking room and constantly tried to get in. She must have been quite confused because she also thought she'd lost her dog. Mum had to tell her that she had found it and that Doctor Tom was looking after it in his flat!

Lots of visitors came and went.

Then – bombshell!! I was transferred to the stroke ward…

Third Stop – Stroke Ward

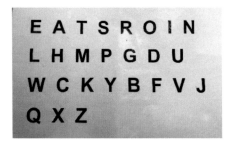

I found myself once again in a single room, with lovely staff. One in particular, who was called Zoe and who was pregnant. The stroke ward was very busy and there were a lot of very sick people, most of them elderly people and quite often dying bodies on trollies went past my window. This is where the speech therapist visited and gave me a spell chart - so my communication began! I was here three weeks.

After I was introduced to my therapist, my communication improved. She taught me how to use eye contact to spell out the words I wished to say. The spell chart was printed onto an A4 piece of paper. It seemed like such an old-fashioned way for mute people to communicate – so basic – to everyone else but I couldn't be more grateful and appreciative of it. This spelling chart would allow me to speak to my loved ones, something I desperately wished for. On numerous occasions, I forgot about my inability to speak: I would look at my family for the answers to questions that I had asked in my head and not out loud… oops.

I admit that at times I would get ridiculously frustrated with myself. I kept forgetting I couldn't speak so people would miss my eye movements and I'd often scream in my head, 'It's the fucking letter A!'.

Rich was the first person to learn my spell chart; it really was unconditional love and he was amazing. We were still together every day and could still have such a laugh. I was even about to spell out, 'Will you marry me?' but something stopped me. I decided not to subject him to this life. At the time, I loved Rich with all my heart and he was the only one for me; I could never even dream about loving anyone else but him. But in the end, I had to let go of my soul mate for his own good. I wanted him to live a great life and not feel as if he was tied down to me because of the condition I was in. Even though he wanted nothing more than to stick by me, I realised that I couldn't offer him the life he deserved. At first, he was insistent that we stay together but I never wanted him to come to resent me or think that I was a burden in the years to come. Sometimes, you have to let those you love fly.

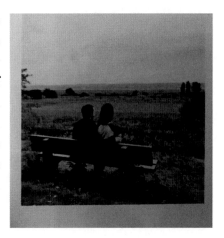

Moving Thumbs

Over the course of time, I managed to teach myself to move different body parts. I would utilise my time each day while my Dad was reading his paper. I would stare and stare at my toes willing them to move.

Please bloody move!

The first thing to move was my thumbs. It was just a flicker but eventually I did the same with my lower arms and various fingers. It was a huge breakthrough; like I was telling everyone, 'I can do this!' and letting them know that I was going to be ok.

One morning, I clearly remember getting the nurse to take my pillow away just before my Dad came in because I wanted to surprise him and show him how I had taught myself to move my neck and turn my head again. He was overwhelmed and I kept going for hours just because I could!

I was so excited by these little triumphs but felt like I had a door slammed in my face time and time again when the doctors would shrug it off and say, 'Oh, it's just a spasm.' I vowed that I would prove them wrong!

Physio

One day, subsequent to my diagnosis, my physiotherapist entered my hospital room with a wheelchair. At that moment, I was overwhelmed; very confused as to why I would need a wheelchair. At first, I assumed that locked-in syndrome was a form of viral infection, however this was not the case. I soon found that I had woken up a completely different person, in a terrifying world. This world seemed rather uncanny; I knew this life had so many similarities, yet I would now be living it differently from the way my life was prior to my accident. The professionals attending to my rare case of locked-in syndrome suggested that I would live a more fulfilling life outside of my bed. I was reassured that a wheelchair would give me some of my independence back in the long run, by allowing me to socialise outside of the hospital and my home. After I came to the realisation of my new life, I felt increasingly devastated, more so than when I initially came out of my coma.

Helplessly, I was later hoisted and gently guided into my wheelchair for a trial, simultaneously surrounded by many doctors and other professionals. I felt so unlike myself and more like a circus freak that I insisted that I had hurt my bottom, meaning I had to be lifted back out of my chair and into bed.

Prison

Hospital is basically an open prison because although it is for your best interests you can't go out of the ward until you have had the OK. I did organise a kind of day-release. This was when I was allowed off the ward but on the doctors' conditions and I had to stay on the hospital site and be back for afternoon medication. The choice of available destinations nearby was pretty limited, but I did my best. I visited the hospice or the care home or the psychiatric building or the oncology ward. Sometimes Mum and I would sunbathe on the grass verge, pretending we were in St Tropez. This must have killed my Mum, but I just had to escape at any chance I could get.

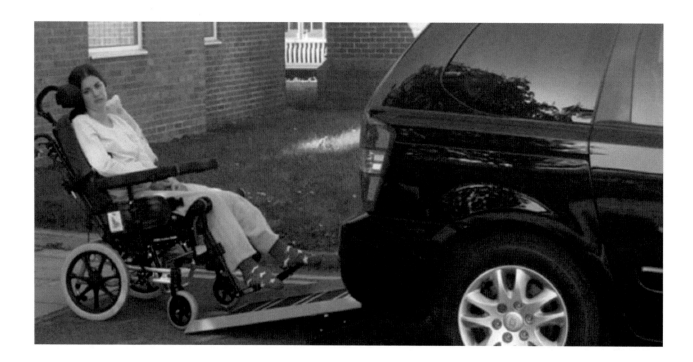

CHAPTER 3

Hospital Two

My fourth stop was the neurological ward at Hospital Two and I was to spend my twenty-first year in neuro rehabilitation here.

I had a nightmare of a journey in the ambulance getting there. It was very distressing, with me crying and my Mum trying not to. I eventually arrived and was shown to my room. It was ok! It was a nice blank canvas and quite spacious. The nurse, Peter, came in to greet me; he was lovely and so kind - such a wonderful guy! He noticed straight away my foot had pressure sores on it; 'I'm going to sort this, Mia, and whilst you are in my care, it will never happen again!'

So, there I was for a year and two weeks.
    Not all good, not all bad...

Day to Day

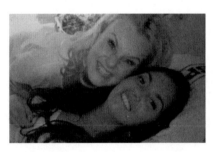

My family, my friend Rich and all my other friends were amazing for the whole year. I never had a day on my own. The hospital staff were fantastic, letting my Dad in from 9-1, then my Mum from 1-7 and Rich and my brother and sister 6.30 - 10/11 every day. Every day my Dad would turn up at the hospital room door with his coffee and paper and we would calmly chat – mostly Dad chatting to me, if we're honest! – and watch the news. From 1pm my Mum, Crazy Caz, would take over and we would go on adventures around the hospital site until the evening where I'd see my sister and brother and Rich. This happened every single day for the duration. So every second I was awake I was never left alone.

The staff also welcomed my friends, letting them into my room at all times. The ward manager, Mark, was totally amazing and enjoyed seeing me with my friends and encouraging me to have mobile beauty treatments with my friend Tash, who is a beautician. She came every week to pamper me and do my nails and wax me, much to the nurses' disapproval. They were livid about the sheets getting wax marks, but hey ho!

Night by Night

So day-to-day life in the hospital was tediously boring, but I'd say that I made the best of it when I could. I would have different visitors every day and see my family but at the end of the day you can't exactly make hospital fun when you're in there for as long as I was.

It was the same basic routine day in and day out and it was hard to shake things up sometimes. The nights were a different story, I would dread them and I would be counting down the hours of daylight in the back of my mind subconsciously; the hours seemed to go on for days, I was alone and absolutely petrified. The night nurses seemed to despise me and made no effort to talk to me or even at me; the lights would go off at 10pm as well as the TVs, and I was left alone with only my own mind to keep me company. I struggled to sleep because it's an inexplicably daunting and distressing position to be in and I would often be awake late into the night.

I have to say these nights were the worst hours of my life.

The mornings were no better, the night staff nearly always got me dressed at 5am because they had to get a certain number of patients ready before they handed over to the day staff. I was nearly always one of the earliest patients to get ready and it really disrupted my sleep even more.

Sign Language

I had to find my fun where I could and there were always funny moments. For example, every afternoon the priest would walk past my room and this one time, Sophie, my Mum and my friend Liv were all in visiting and he collared us. He started talking to me in sign language and everyone was on their knees laughing too hard to tell him I wasn't deaf.

Memory

I remember one day testing my memory, things like where I lived and my house and phone number. I did this because I presumed that I had been left brain damaged. I did find it difficult to remember these things at first – I couldn't even remember what had happened to me; about the accident and why I was in hospital.

During a stroke, the brain is damaged, so it was possible that I would have difficulty concentrating, and experience short-term memory problems, depending on which areas of the brain have been damaged. Some stroke patients find that it is difficult to learn new things or have problems remembering things from long ago because it is hard to find the information that the brain has stored – the old ways of finding that information have been lost. Sometimes things improve or stroke patients learn strategies to cope with memory loss. I wanted to find out whether I could remember the things that were important to me. I discovered that in fact my memory wasn't badly affected and I found that I could remember things and also learn new things in just the same way as I had before the stroke.

Feeding Tube

I had to have this horrific operation to put a feeding tube into my tummy and I woke up mid operation. Blurry faces and bright lights. I've never felt pain like it. All I could taste was banana anesthetic, I don't even like bananas!!! Initially, I was fed via a tube up my nose, then they fed me via an overnight drip. Then I went to three meal-replacement drinks and a pure calorie shot, which was fed to me through my PEG feeding tube (short for percutaneous endoscopic gastrostomy), directly into my stomach. They were intended to help me to put on weight because I had lost so much while I was in a coma. Then I went to eating orally again; initially Weetabix and two shakes, then Weetabix and yoghurt and two shakes. Gradually, I threw in any food I could get my hands on. Sure, it's been a long gruelling process, 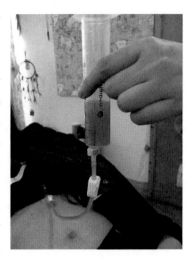 but man has it been worth it because now I'm on three solid meals per day and appreciate and savour every mouthful, as when I was in hospital I'd daydream about all the different foods I'd have.

Nurses

Relatively soon after the stroke, I had regained my character and, just like before, I had my own opinions and judgements. I quickly sussed out which nurses were good and which ones were 'bad'. Of course, there wasn't much I could do to show when I was annoyed but my trick was to purposely laugh as hard as I could when a nurse I didn't like was by me, so that my chocolate milk would spill everywhere and they would have to clear it up!

Reputation

I had quite the reputation as the mischievous one, but I wasn't going to lie down and feel sorry for myself, and my friends and family and I had as much fun as possible. Me and my best friend Olivia would go out in the snow and my other best friend Kate, would give me melted chocolate. All the boys who are really close friends, would come and cause absolute carnage, me and Mum would go to the Oncology ward for days out and me and Sophie would wind everyone right up! I had also met my 'neighbours' on the ward. They annoyed the hell out of me and kept me awake, so I would get my friend to put on my Clubland CD full blast at times when they finally wanted to rest themselves. I certainly found ways to express myself, even if I couldn't shout at them!

Phil

I only met one friend in hospital, he was called Phil and he had a brain tumour. We became inseparable. You would think during my time I'd meet lots of people but Phil and I had this connection and got each other; he would turn up to my room and make me laugh so much. Phil was such an unlikely friend as he was much older, but when I first met him, we passed each other in the hallway in the hospital, stopped and smiled at each other. I think Phil could see that I was unable to speak, so he would greet me with a great big smile. I could see his menacing behaviour written on his face and this was when I knew we could be friends. I felt so amazing that I had met someone that I could be friends with, we were so similar, we shared the same humour and characteristics, but eventually after making this friendship that carried me through my long sentence in the hospital, I was unaware that I was about to have my heart ripped out right from my chest...

My only friend in this horrible place was gone.
    I got my Mum to push me to his room but there was no sign of him.
    No Phil? None of his belongings?

My Mum asked a nurse where he was and they replied the local nursing home. I was absolutely gutted but more importantly I thought, 'Surely this was planned and so why didn't anyone tell me this to prepare me?' I was certainly old enough.

Mum kindly took me to the nursing home where Phil was. As soon as I entered the premises I was overwhelmed by the dark atmosphere. The place also stunk. I suddenly panicked, I was wondering whether this was the plan for every patient.

This was the last time I'd ever see Phil because he died and I was lost without my partner in crime.

I partly keep up my menacing behaviour to keep his legacy going.

It was a long year, but after a few attempts to get home to visit with lifts arranged by charities and in taxis, (which was kind of them but horrendous for me) by magic a slinky black car appeared. It was a Kia, that had been adapted to my needs. My friends, Mike Greenacre and Sue Jones, had organised a massive fundraiser in Manchester, plus my Mum and Dad had just bought a new car and so had I, before the stroke, so all the money was put together and bingo! I had a new lifeline. So now I could escape from Hospital Two, go shopping, which I had really missed, and go home for a few hours. Wow! That made such a difference.

The nurses there (apart from two, who we will not mention) had been utterly amazing. They enjoyed coming into my room and chatting; such kindness. We had such good laughs. On the other hand, when I say I had a tough time in hospital it couldn't be more true. The days were fine but I would dread the clock in my room hitting 10pm. If I needed anything, I had a buzzer I could use but one of the regular nurses would walk into my room, turn my buzzer off and go out again. So, I'd cry myself to sleep every night without fail, fearing what could happen in the night with no one to shout for if I needed them. No one thought this could be true until one morning my Dad came into my room to find my buzzer had been taken away from me. We were even thinking seriously about fitting hidden cameras. I wish we had because only I will ever know how badly I was treated at times. There were other things, like the nurses mispronouncing my name as 'My-ah', much to my annoyance. Of course, I couldn't easily let them know how I felt, but it got so bad that my sister went wild and they were in no doubt after that. The good thing is that these experiences only made me realise how wonderful, kind and dedicated the majority of the nurses really are. It certainly helped me to see the good in most people who are so different from these few by comparing their behaviour.

CHAPTER 4

Final Destination

A lot of time passed. Days at the hospital turned into months, and the next thing I knew it was Christmas Day. It was positively the worst Christmas ever! Picture an undecorated hospital room and everyone piled in and sat on plastic chairs. I found having my first Christmas/Mothers' Day/Easter and birthday in hospital horrific, though the staff were amazing – even buying me gifts. It felt so lonely, even though I was surrounded by family and friends.

Aiming to go Home

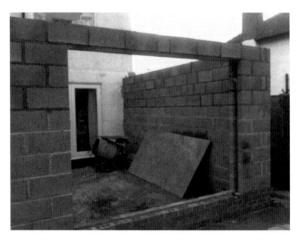

By now I was determined to get home. Among the hospital staff there was even talk of putting me in a care home but my Dad had arranged a local builder to kindly build my palace – an extension to be added to the house – and I spent a considerable amount of time planning my new rooms at home. This was my only glimmer of hope. Every day my Dad and I would sit in my hospital room and plan the layout and decoration and the first day they let me out for two hours I went to B and Q and chose my paint! Now that I had the car, we could go out and choose things like the colour schemes and furniture. I was able to come home on day visits and enjoyed watching the builders at work and my room taking shape.

On my birthday, I organised a party at the local golf club, which was fantastic and a good opportunity for everyone to celebrate with me. It was great with the singing sensation Tom Spence DJ-ing and singing and my sister Sophie singing too. But I had to go back to my cell that evening; that was really hard.

Now though my mission was to get home. It sounds easy – the extension was done, everything was in place, my care package, my room and I'd had a trial run of staying overnight with carers. However, Health and Social Services couldn't agree on my funding. I was stuck! It was awful!

Paperwork

I met my first social worker one day and was so excited at the prospect of coming home, but little did I know I was a long way off because I had a mound of paperwork; it was just false hope every time. I needed to feel like my sentence would soon be over, and I'd be brought back to reality. My family fought every day for months for the hospital to let me home. The Primary Care Commission had a big argument about whether I 'belonged' to the Health Service to fund my being at home or Social Services. Why did they think it was OK to play piggy-in-the-middle with me? How these people sleep at night, I don't understand!

First Fundraiser

In December 2010, a year after my stroke, I organised a fundraiser for the neurology ward, which was held at The Thatch pub in the Raby-mere. The pub staff were brilliant; providing free food. Sophie and our friend Matt provided the entertainment, the night was fantastic and I raised £1,500 pounds. I bought PlayStations, game consoles and TVs with DVD players for single rooms in the hospital.

Leaving Hospital

It was literally my worst nightmare to be stuck in hospital for so long. I've always been hospital phobic and would actually faint when I was younger and attended routine appointments. I've got slightly better but I don't much want to be going near hospitals anytime soon.

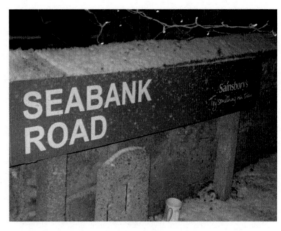

After nine months of feeling institutionalised, they had at least started to talk about me leaving the hospital. Still I was a prisoner. Then finally on Christmas Eve 2010, after lots of begging and furious phone calls, Health decided to finance me. I was going home: my sentence was up!

One day, I was lying in my hospital bed staring at my wall of photos of my previous life waiting for my Dad to appear at 8am and he didn't arrive.

Suddenly my Mum bounded through the door; I was so confused. But lo and behold, big changes were about to unfold.

My house was ready. And the reason my Dad hadn't turned up was because he had the meeting with the care agency manager to assess any risks at my house. BUT she took one foot through the door and she stated, 'There's no chance that Mia is returning home just yet.' To which my Dad desperately replied, 'Would you be able to come back at 9am tomorrow please?'

The word got around my street that that I was unable to come home as my newly-built house extension was not yet ready. Later, I was so overwhelmed to find that the whole road had pulled together as a community to finish my house.

Rich did the electrics and his best friend did the plumbing, working right through the night. Graham, my next-door neighbour, was steam cleaning while Lynn and John were making the cupboards. Other neighbours did the tiling and Jen and Sarah, my neighbours, and my sister were putting together the finishing touches; also Jenny and Roger were moving the furniture and Heather and Ian brought round a huge lasagne and a box of beer for everyone. The next morning the woman arrived and my room was like a miracle transformation. The manager looked surprised and said to my Dad, 'Mr Austin, your daughter is coming home.'

Coming home was the thing I wanted most.

I didn't necessarily care about what had happened to me as my friends and family had reassured me that everything was going to be OK, and we could get through it together.

And my wish came true, on the Christmas Eve my Mum came to see me at a random time and burst out to me, 'You're coming home, Mimi". I spelt out AMAZING, but deep down inside I thought that there was a slim chance that I would be going home as I had had so many false positives about returning home for months. I didn't want to build my hopes up, but my Mum said, 'TODAY, YOU'RE COMING HOME TODAY!'

I think I experienced every emotion. I was absolutely ecstatic, and I think my eyes popped out of my head and I sobbed tears of happiness. Out came my family, armed with bin bags to frantically pack my belongings before anyone could stop the great escape. Was I dreaming again?

This was it. Dr. Hughes, my consultant, and the favourites Annie, Chris and Mary were all there to wave me goodbye. Then the girls from the pharmacy came with a goodbye present; there wasn't a dry eye in the house. That was the end of the bad times.

On the return home I took the opportunity to appreciate every little thing around me from the smell of the sea salt in the air to the smell of the Comfort on my bedding at home. I finally returned home and so many memories rushed back to me; the house my sister was born in on the living room carpet... a place I thought I would never see again. But I was back where I belonged.

I came home!!

Little did I know that my Mum's friend had entered me, my family and our road into the Sainsbury's Christmas competition – and we had won! The street had been transformed with snow, lights, reindeer, Santa, carol singers and food and drink, followed by a spectacular firework display. It was magical! It was a massive thank you to our wonderful neighbours, who had all pitched in on getting my extension ready.

Five Wishes

I really wish five things:

1. That the doctors had taken me seriously when I went to the GP, complaining of persistent migraines.
2. That during the initial examination the doctors could have diagnosed the stroke a lot faster.
3. I wish I could have been sent straight to Hospital Two.
4. And I feel strongly that I should have been granted physio under the National Health Service from day one of being home, because I feel any initial support would have got me moving, rather than wasting four years until I was able to afford private physio.
5. What I'd give to have one last argument with my sister about something petty.

Attitudes and Perspectives

Everything has changed!

After waking up from my coma, it was like I had woken up ten years later. It seemed like there were a lot more problems in the world after I woke up, or maybe I just had a different perspective on life. I had never been so grateful to be alive, I became more aware of the smallest inconveniences that people would complain about, they just seemed to unimportant to me. I have never once felt sorry for myself but when there are people complaining about the smallest things I just think to myself, 'Look at what happened to me, why are you complaining?'. When I come across people acting like the world is going to end because they have broken a nail, I think, 'Get a grip. We have homeless people starving and people dying fighting for their countries! Shut up!'

I feel like I went to sleep leaving everything peaceful and society changed so much by the time I woke up and came round. Initially, it was small things like people's hair colours changing or everyone was driving white cars and they were all absolutely glued to their iPhones. In fact, I tried so much to fit in, I got the iPad and in occupational therapy every day I tried to learn how to use it, with a stylus in my mouth, but I couldn't get my head to move so I gave up.

All my separate friendship groups had come together, my little sister had swapped jobs and Mum and Dad retired early, so it was all changes around me. I even had my cousin Kate feeding me chocolate until I got caught by a nurse who confiscated my stash – I didn't realise that I couldn't really eat at that stage.

My impression was that world politics was quiet when I left and I came back to terrorism at its peak and what was most scary was to learn how much of a mess the health service was in, especially when I was spending every waking minute in their hands.

Education and Politics

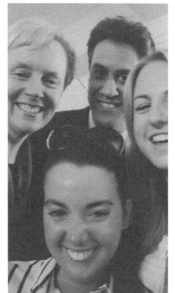

I'm not sure what you know about senses but they say that as you lose one sense, you gain another. In my case, not only had I missed out on what was going on in the world around me, I compensated by getting hugely into politics. I went to see Ed Miliband giving a speech nearby. I had become more intelligent to what was going on and the figures were getting absorbed into my memory.

I like watching crime documentaries and my Dad is in to crime books; also, one of my carers is doing a degree in criminology so we were speaking about that and I started up looking up courses. Eventually, I did a criminology course at a local college and went onto do a forensics online course with the Open University.

So much has changed including me. I developed coping mechanisms. There isn't much to it; you either sink or you swim. In the first few years, I wrote a lot of poetry because it took my mind off the frustration. I had got myself involved so much in the idea of travelling that I educated myself about how different countries lived and their cultures and religions.

Home

And so I came home. My new bedroom is fully adapted, but you wouldn't know apart from the ramp outside. I don't have any equipment on show and my hospital bed has been painted and is decorated like a day bed. I have room to have everything as normal as possible and the carers are two steps away in a gorgeous decorated room with a TV and big chairs and fridge, a kettle, toaster etc. I also have a wet room.

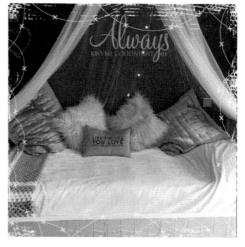

The first few days home were the best! I thought to myself, maybe I'm not unlucky that this has happened to me, I'm lucky in a strange way, because it has made me appreciate absolutely everything more. It was so great to see everyone and then it was the district nurse appointments and wheelchair centre appointments every day and I soon came to realise that I hated all of this. I'd gone from being a really private person to having files written about me, with details about every meal, my weight, my skin, what I've said, my house layout, the risks; the nurses just thought they held the rights to my body and checked my skin every few days! I also had to go to a meeting every month, where the big wigs would argue about the ins and outs of my care. To start with I had emergency carers, who called in for 15 minutes, three times a day and then the main ones started.

CHAPTER 5

The Start of Me

Mia's Angels began and this was the start of me. I now had the funding for my very own personal health budget for 24 hours every day. I could hire the nice carers and sack the freaks; I could do my own routines and adapt them to have certain people working according to my plans. I finally had control over my life and it was just the beginning. I did so much stuff that I couldn't do before and was immediately happier and had so much fun. Being a manager at 24 was of course very difficult to adjust to but I love to organise and be there for my carers, just like they are there for me.

Mountains for Mia – June 2010 Three Peaks Challenge

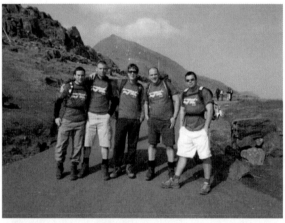

Living in the hospital was driving me crazy. I desperately wanted to return home but in order to be able to live there comfortably I needed some work done to the house, which comes at a price!

I only had bit of savings so had no more money, and my Mum and Dad had had to retire.

Rich and my brother Sam knew how much I wanted to be at home again and were determined to get me there. On top of working full times jobs and coming to see me every day, they put all of their effort into organising an enormous charity event based on what they both do best... mountain climbing!

They decided on the Three Peak Challenge and called the event 'Mountains for Mia', getting all the lads they knew to join in with them. Loads of other people stepped up to help too, all for little old me! Rich and Sam would put every spare minute they had into planning and promoting the event, they planned everything down to the smallest detail and even designed and made T-shirts and wristbands especially for the day.

    I couldn't actually believe that people went to these lengths to help me out and that they raised thousands. Everyone I knew climbed the last mountain and the fittest of the bunch did all three. At the end of the challenge everyone was dripping with sweat and covered head to toe in mud but to celebrate their success in completing the day we had a BBQ at the end.

I can't actually give this gesture the justice and credit it deserves, we ended up raising the much-needed funds that meant I could move back home at last. I have had many people fundraise for me but the most important was the Three Peaks Challenge. The money raised changed my life from that moment to this day. Essentially it paid for me to come home because the government grant would only have paid for us to install a bathroom on the ground floor at home.

The Santa Dash – December annually

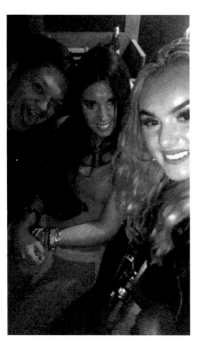

The second biggest thing has been the Heswall Santa Dash, which is a pub crawl organised by a close friend of mine, Rob, and my sister Sophie. One night each year, my hometown is filled by a sea of people willing to purchase tickets for a night out where 100 percent of the ticket money goes to charity. Every pub and bar in Heswall goes all out in order to provide for their target audience, things such as snow machines have been used to attract more people. My organisation, Mountains for Mia, was chosen to receive the money that was raised. It is an extremely overwhelming sentiment, something that I am very appreciative of and taken aback by each time. So much effort is put into this event in order to help me live a better life; the staff of the venues completely stress themselves out in order to get as much money raised as possible. However, ultimately the praise lies with Rob and Sophie, who go to such lengths in order for this event to be successful. Without sounding ungrateful, it is nice to be reminded that you're not forgotten when Christmas time comes around. This event not only reinforces the community spirt of my hometown, but also enables me to do many things that I wouldn't be able to do without the charity money; without this I wouldn't be able to pay the bills for my half of the house. The money is put towards my rehabilitation, including physio, hydrotherapy, salt therapy, oxygen therapy and acupuncture. I also have to fund little things that the NHS cannot provide for me. These things include hand and foot splints.

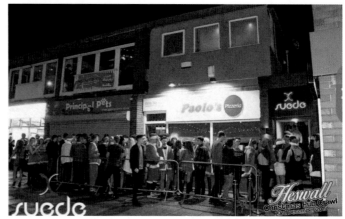

Adopt-a-nan

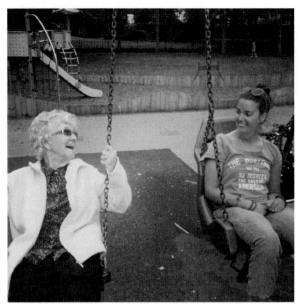

Back home, I also adopted a nan; her name was Rose and every week I'd take her shopping or to garden centres, with Karen driving my slinky Kia. She really appreciated the company, as her family wanted nothing to do with her. We would sit and plan a list of everything she wanted to do and we did it. We had a scream together; she loved me and I loved her and she would put cigarettes in my mouth but one day I heard that she'd had a fall. I went to visit her in hospital and that very night she died but I knew that I'd made her very happy.

I have recently adopted another nan; my Mum's friend's mother. Her name is Margaret, she's is 85 and living alone. While she does have a son and daughter, they each have families and can only free up a couple days in the week between them. It can be lonely around the winter time, especially for older people, so I'm trying to help where I can. Each week I spend a few hours with Margaret to keep her company. She is a very interesting person with so many funny stories to tell. I love spending time with her, but what I love more is that I know she's never going to be lonely while I'm around. It is fate that I now see her because her granddaughter Charlotte once ran the Edinburgh marathon for me and raised a huge amount.

Mia's Angels

I've had some odd carers but my current team are the best lot. They are a range of different ages and all have different talents. The first lot of carers were really good and they helped me see that not everyone in the profession was bad, but as the company manager got to know me, she shoved any old carer at me. Unfortunately for her, I still got on well with them! It really did seem that she tried to make life difficult for me. This got worse over the next 18 months, but karma did its job; I was the first person in my area given a personal health budget and everything changed. I was so much happier and had a new sense of responsibility for my own

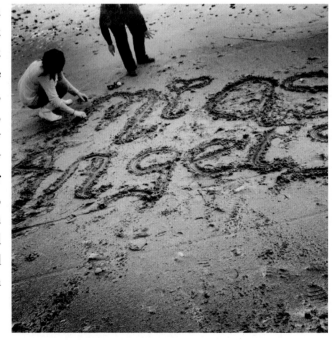

care, including hiring and interviewing, and organising training for the carers. The carers who have worked with me have varied – some, I've wondered why I let them through the front door, right to the best of the best.

Karen has been with me since day one of my care team, for eight years in total. She is the cement and my guru. Karen is the one that takes me on holiday and even takes me on her own family holidays. We went to the Bob Marley Festival and I have been go-karting with her. She is the one that cares for people when they are ill. Her kids are like my cousins. Her boyfriend and kids even came with me on my biggest adventure – to Thailand. She is a real rock and is always there when I need her, day or night, she is the foundation of Mia's Angels.

Lesley is cray-cray but she brightens the day-day! She might be crazy but she's been with me now for over four years and is amazing at her job. I think she just gets me. She's a very positive human and it rubs off on everyone. She knows how to take control of a situation and resolve it to keep our days running smoothly and trouble free. She will put music on and dance around my room and get up to lots of other antics that make me howl with laughter. Lesley shows so much empathy towards me and fusses over me when I'm feeling a little low or when I am ill. She has the ability to put a good spin on anything. I can trust her with my life, I can also leave my paperwork with her when I'm ill, with no doubt that it will be sorted for me.

Han makes me smile. She joined Mia's Angels about four years ago and since then she has well and truly evolved into one of my best angels. She is head of the night staff because she has the ability to keep a personal yet professional relationship. She has the ability to lighten any room with joy and laughter, and since I met her we have become close friends. I look forward to seeing her when she comes to work. Hannah brings out the best in me; whenever she believes I am being difficult she will be straight with me and help me with sorting a situation. As we are close in age, me and Hannah can see each other's point of view and understand where we are both coming from. Every night shift, she would get my biggest smile and we would laugh hysterically at everything.

Jess is the youngest carer. She joined Mia's Angels at the age of sixteen, four years ago. Even though she is the youngest member of my team, she is extremely mature for her age. She really does take the best care of me as she knows me so well, she can just guess what I am thinking. We are ten years apart, but it's like we're twins... we are both fashion and makeup crazy and we have everything in common, from humour to liking the same films.

Sophie Loyns has been with me for just over a year, she is one of the sweetest people I've ever met; she is so kind and caring, making her a vital member of Mia's Angels. I feel so lucky to have her looking after me as she knows exactly what I want, when I want it. She has a lovely, bubbly personality and always sees the good in me. She is a such a natural when it comes to fulfilling her role as a carer, as she's such a caring person.

Beckie has been with me for a year and a half, but since joining Mia's Angels she has maintained a role that could not be replaced. At first, she seems a little quiet but then you get through to the bubbly, lovely and funny Beck. Since being introduced to Beckie, she has inspired me to go bigger and beyond what people think I can do. She seen potential in me to be a better me; she even inspired me to go to college to continue my education. We've both studied a similar course, which I love and I am now excelling in. She goes beyond her working hours, and even comes in on a day off to braid my hair. Every night we have such a laugh together.

Lorraine is one of my cutest angels, with a very kind and caring heart. She has been with me for nearly three years and has always taken such good care of me and has always pushed me to pursue my dreams. Lorraine and I have travelled together all the way to Gambia. She is a very smiley and positive person and can always cheer me up with her presence.

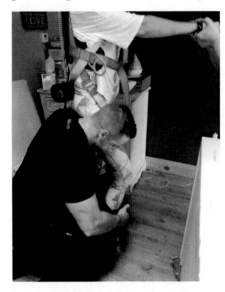

The relationship I have with Mike is like one from the films; he is like a pocketful of sunshine. He makes me smile from 8am till 10pm. He makes me get up and dressed and go out and we do everything together. We text all day, every day; unless we are already out at the pub. He has been with me for a year and a half but will stay in my heart for forever and a day.

Over the years, I've seen a few private physios, as I'm unbelievably not entitled to any NHS physio at all. I was at the gym one afternoon, showing my Mum around, and Mum being Mum was off talking to the guy at reception. That guy turned out to be Mark. He was working as a personal trainer and offered to help me. My first session, all I could do was stand up. Since then he has helped me so much with lots of time and different therapies to help me get to where I am today. He later quit his job as a personal trainer and came to work for me doing night shifts he has been with me for the past three years. Mark went on to do physiotherapy at college and university. He also volunteers at the oxygen centre I go to and continues to do the gym and physio with me on his days off. I know from this he sounds like a saint but he has become a good friend.

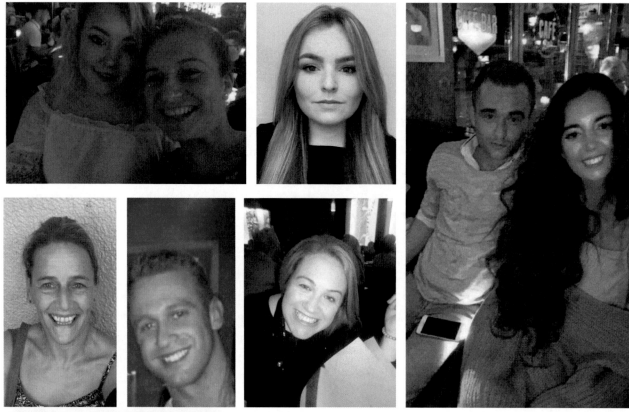

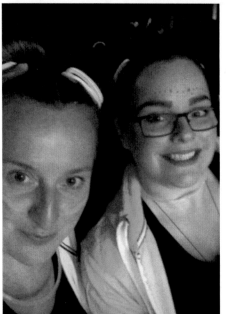

These people are my support network. My family and friends without a doubt are the glue; my friends are true friends and I've erased the fake friends from my life because I don't need them. My carers support me every day as well; I have met some of the nicest people and also some of the worst.

Family

The stroke must have affected my family in a huge way. My Dad was a head teacher and my Mum was the head of drama and they both had to retire. My brother, Sam, is a quiet guy and is still very quiet about it all and my sister just takes it in her stride now but I imagine at the time of the accident they must have been distraught. Now we have so much family time together and we make more of an effort to visit relatives and communicate; after all my family are my life.

Friends

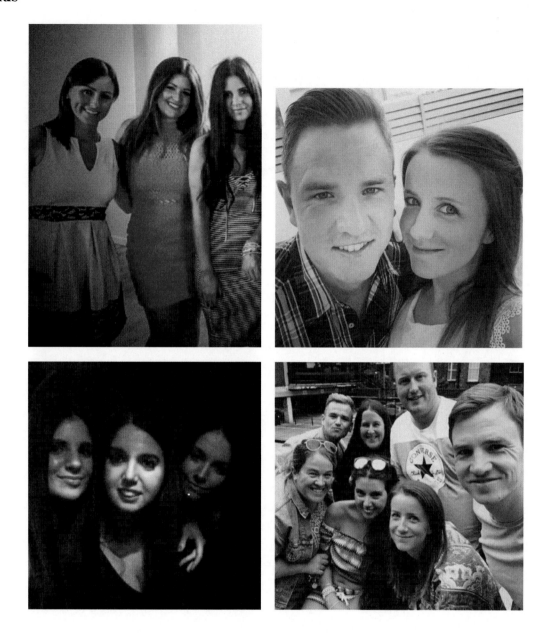

They say you don't know your true friends until something happens to you. This couldn't be more true. At the start every Tom, Dick and Harry came in to see me for their conscience and many have never bothered with me since, but my real friends have always been there for me and I love them all so much. They have given me so many amazing memories and they have definitely kept me going. It is lovely that my personal assistants have become friends as well. My best friend is my sister, she is just my mini-me and you are sisters by blood but friends by choice; we get each other and bounce off each other and can literally have a conversation just using our eyes and she is telepathic. It is great!

CHAPTER 6

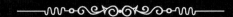
Changes in Me

At first, I worried about what I would turn out like, but I don't actually know because I've gone totally the opposite. I lost my confidence in hospital; in fact, for the first year I refused to even look in the mirror because I was so scared to see what I'd look like; I thought a stroke made one side of your face droop and taking photo was totally out of the question. Recently I've gone to another level and won't even have a photo in the wheelchair, or if I do the carers have to crop it out after. Of course, I'm quieter but my eyes speak volumes. I'm a lot feistier but I have to be because in hospital I kept quiet and look what happened! I'm definitely more daring but what can be scarier? I also have a much more positive outlook on life. Only positive changes have occurred really.

My new-life resolution

One day I was put in front of the TV and I thought, 'Why should I be subjected to this lifestyle? Hell no!'

I got my computer and researched adrenaline activities. I think you definitely go in to one of two directions when you're ill; you either get really depressed and don't move from the house, thinking that this life will never get better or you go out and do crazy things to better your life experience, participate in crazy activities and at that moment I decided that this is exactly the way my life is going.

Stepping Up

I'm forever watching the way people move so I can figure out how to do it myself, including walking, sitting down and getting up because I've figured out once I see how to do everything and remind myself how to do everything and remind my brain how to do everything, it will know how to do it. I used to do a lot of dancing and gymnastics when I was younger but I don't mind not being able to move again to that extent, I just care about simple movements. I've never stopped trying and I never will.

Equipment

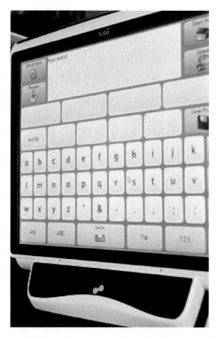

I spent my first three years after the accident using just a spell chart and thanks to my Dad's research he found out about Tobii Dynavox Eyegaze computer, which has been a lifeline for me. I only have it due to the massive fundraising efforts of my supporters and I'm very grateful. It allows me to 'type' out messages and much more, just using my eyes to indicate a position on a computer screen. I've written this whole book myself using it! Although my eyes do strain from using it so much, I don't wear glasses; I'm just sensible and when my eyes get tired I don't use it or use the rest button to switch off. The company is Swedish and are award winning and have moved on technology by about twenty years.

Whoever invented the Tobii Dynavox for people who are unable to speak is beyond intelligent. I don't speak at all apart from the odd word like 'no' and 'ow' and I didn't know such things existed before but now they are the only way I can communicate without getting frustrated. It also works by scanning my eyes and the technology has skipped centuries since Stephen Hawking's', so I don't sound anything like him. If I am out, I can either use my tablet version or anyone I go out with can spell manually because they have all memorised my spell chart. I use a lot of social media accounts from my computer and email, text, calculator, calendar etc., basically like a phone.

I don't really have a view on limiting others' screen time, it's their life; if they choose not to use their common sense then they have to accept the consequences.

So gradually I got very tiny movements back. Initially I was assigned this massive, cumbersome bog-standard wheelchair, but I chose not to have a wheelchair; to take the ugly foot plates off; to take the headrest off and to shave the sides of my chair off and to support myself. The physios would never ever say you can do without these things so it proves, if you don't do it yourself, things will never improve. Eventually I had a chair that's specifically moulded to my shape by a company called S.O.S. (Specialised Orthotic Services). They are brilliant with me and adapt it with me in mind. Respecting that I'm still young and vain, they will shave off parts, so it's not noticeable. I have a hospital profile bed with a pressure mattress, but me being me, I got my Dad and neighbour Neil to paint it all and disguise the sides so it looks like a chic daybed. I haven't got any other assistive technology.

My Visitor from the Isle of Man

I stupidly asked my consultant one day whether I would be able to meet someone else my age with locked-in syndrome. He brought someone over from the Isle of Man to Hospital Two. He was absolutely lovely, but I really wish I hadn't requested to meet him because it made me really self-conscious. I was even more reluctant to look in the mirror.

Social Media – a Mixed Blessing

Social media is a difficult topic, as I rely on it both as a blog and personally for my independence. There are two sides to social media; I find it a great way to keep people updated on my progress and it's equally rewarding when people comment on how well I've done. I use my Eyegaze computer to communicate with people on social media; I use it to update my Mountains for Mia blog to keep people updated on my progress and also to help others in my situation and for people to keep up with my many adventures and learn about my fundraising projects. I use Facebook mainly; it's also a way I can keep up to date with others who maybe I don't see as often as I would like. Also, I rely on Facebook Messenger to communicate with everyone with daily messages; it's how I can organise my days. I don't know where I would be without it as I don't have texts.

On the flip side, social media can be invasive and used in a horrible way. I remember the first time I went on my Facebook account after the stroke and saw that people had written 'rest in peace' on my wall and people thought I had actually died. That was horrific! I have had experience of people pretending to be me and using my photos on Facebook. One ex-carer wrote nasty things about me on Facebook and another pretended to be me on Snapchat by using my pictures and created a whole profile, where she added my friends and started talking to them. These were very distressing incidents so, perhaps more than most people, I need social media in my life but I have to be very careful when using it as I can be a victim of the bad side of it.

Money

I am so thankful that, prior to the stroke, I'd been saving for my mortgage. I know it's crap that I didn't have the chance to get my house but it's a blessing that I've still benefited from my money and been able to travel. Being stupid – bungee-ing and swimming with sharks – but that's how I've chosen to use it.

Therapies

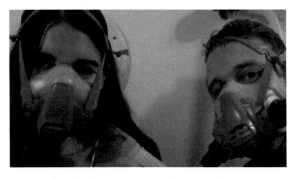

Every week I try to do one day in the gym with Mark, which is extremely hard work. Not physically but my brain feels like it's going to explode! One time I even burst capillaries in my eyes because I tried so hard. I also try and swim one day with Mark, which again is mentally draining but it's so much easier to move because the water supports me. I also do oxygen therapy, which is also draining and also causes pain in my ears due to the pressure but I know it's good for me, and salt theraphy, also known as Halotheraphy,which is proven to help with respiratory problems and is helping lots with my reoccurring chest infections. For years it seemed that I didn't qualify for NHS physio, which was the most ridiculous thing and very distressing to me, that I'd been written off and given up on. I'm really motivated to improve, so that I can carry on my adventures and my fundraising. The latest news is that the NHS will fund my physio; I have every hope that this will come about and aim to improve even more.

Christmas present

On Christmas Eve of 2015, Mark and I had a planned a very special surprise for my family. They had all been told by doctors that I would never walk again, but I do like to prove doctors wrong! So I had been working on taking steps in water for months and Christmas Eve was show time. We told everyone to meet us at the swimming pool…

My family had no idea what to expect when they arrived at the pool; they had no idea what Mark and I had been up to and their jaws dropped to the floor when they watched me walk two whole lengths of the pool. Words couldn't begin to explain how happy they were and their gratitude to Mark; this was the best Christmas present they could dream of!

Stroke Centre Plan

Every week, I got by on physio and speech therapy and got that tiny bit stronger. I decided that when I'm better I'm going to set up my own stroke centre with TVs and bright colours and physio rooms with loud music where friends can visit at any time. Me and my friend Mark have this dream to set up our own stroke rehabilitation centre one day: I would run it and he is going to do the physio and we also want to buy a portable oxygen xpod, a system that allows you to monitor your oxygen levels without needles.

Eating

I mentioned that I had surgery to have my feeding tube put in fairly early on. I still have it now and use it for water and medication. I can eat orally now, I just take my time. I eat everything, although technically I should have soft foods. After getting pneumonia last year, I was told I could no longer have water orally through a syringe and so now I can only use small, lollypop-style sponges to moisten my mouth. Luckily, I can still have alcohol – hell, yeah!

CHAPTER 7

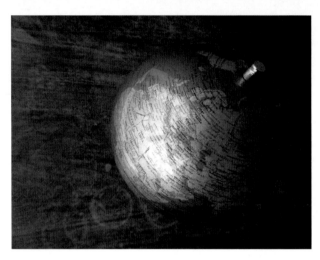

Travelling

Getting from place to place has been a distressing concept for me ever since the stroke; feeling so helpless. Once I physically got stuck going from one hospital to another and being hospital phobic makes things worse. Nevertheless, I live now to travel it keeps me going although it really, really hurts my bum sitting, especially on a plane, but I can see through the pain knowing adventure is waiting.

Dreams

Everyone has dreams – right? So why can't I have mine?

I don't have locked-in syndrome; I have something far more complex, called locked-in-the-UK syndrome. I dream every day about moving abroad, the warmth on my muscles, no worries but whether to have mango or strawberries and the sound of waves and happy people rather than carers flicking the kettle on. But it's never going to happen because the doctors, specialists, district nurses and dieticians all have a massive hold on me, as well as the NHS who hold the funding for my 24-hour care.

Still a Geek

I am a geek; I love educating myself further. I think it's really important to keep the brain active so I go to college and I'm studying criminal justice. I also watch so many documentaries, mainly on my idol Stacey Dooley, who travels and makes a documentary. I also love Reggie Yates documentaries and various documentaries on neuroplasticity and the way the brain adapts after injury; it's so interesting. I also have really got into politics and even attended a speech by Ed Miliband, meeting him afterwards.

Help, I Have a Carrot on my Lung!

I knew I would eventually get pneumonia, I just thought maybe at the age of 80. It was horrific the night I got rushed to hospital; I was just repeatedly sick and fainted lots. My chest felt like ice. It was a good lesson to keep myself warm and I've since looked at the vitamins and supplements I take and I've slowed down on the nights out (a bit). Unfortunately, it's taken me back about two years on my physio progress but I can do that again. I played a trick on the doctor... I opened the window next to me and took the covers off, so that my temperature would drop right down and they could discharge me. At this point I had to stop drinking, which sucks. I now have the tiniest bits of water from a useless little sponge.

Holidays

Following my own motto, I live my life and I live to travel. It's true that people thought I was crazy going to such dangerous places. Strangely, though, when my family took me travelling around Thailand I have to say that was the most normal I've been treated. People say the last place you should go in a wheelchair is the souks of Marrakesh but I did this too – and even rode a camel. Here are my adventures so far.

Florida – June 2012

I was excited to go to Florida and it was an amazing holiday, but it got off to a bad start. When I was getting off the plane, after a nine hour grueling plane journey, the flight attendants dropped me trying to pick me off the seat, OWCH!!! I landed right on the plane floor, in front of everyone on the flight. Obviously, I was in a lot of pain and I was extremely distressed, due to shock. I already felt as if my holiday was ruined. Florida was a regular holiday as we didn't have much of an adventure and, without wanting to be ungrateful, I feel like all ill people typically go to Disney and it shouldn't have to be that way. This is probably why I decided I was just going to push all boundaries and not simply do the usual things that any person in my situation might do. Months and years of doing what was expected of me, of being a (relatively) well-behaved patient for the good of my health had built up a bubble inside me and it had burst - it was at this stage I started to rebel...

Newquay – 2012

I went to Newquay in 2012. I needed a break and after my trip to Florida, which I found so difficult, I wanted to stay in the UK. I drove to a gorgeous little house in Newlyn with my family and carers. I still had to look after myself and stay warm, so I hadn't yet tried any adrenaline sports at this time. The week was just what I needed. I visited all the local attractions, including the Eden Project, and spent time at the beach where Sophie and my Dad went surfing. I went onto the beach and got stuck! Luckily, after attempting to move, some very helpful young men who were surfing came running over and carried me off the beach. It's times like this that being in a wheelchair has its advantages.

Spain – 2014

This was my first holiday abroad with my own carers; I went with them and my Mum, Dad and sister to a gorgeous hotel in Alcudia in Spain. At this point I was as well as I am now and hadn't even been in a swimming pool. Our hotel was right by the sea and I took a huge, inflatable lounge chair to relax on. It was so hot and for the first time I went in the pool with the help of my Dad. We visited the beaches, went in the sea, visited old Alcudia and just relaxed; it was amazing to spend some quality time with my family. It was here that I discovered my love for chocolate crêpes.

Gambia – October 2015

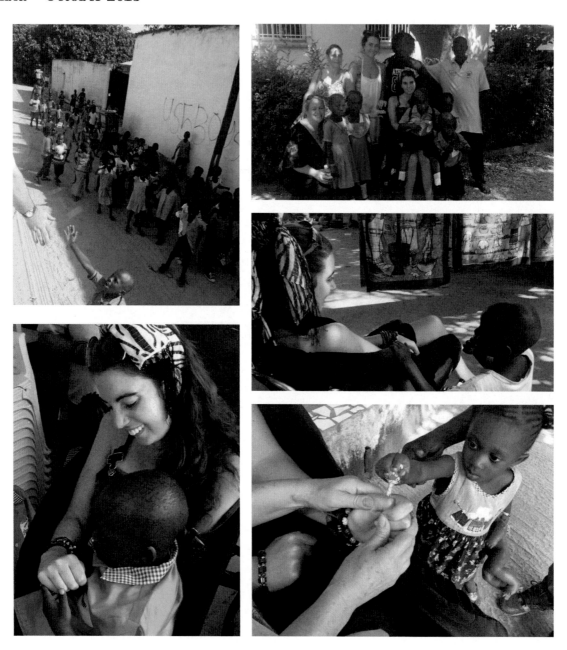

Where do I start? Gambia was one of the most amazing and different experiences I have ever had, even to this day it still stands as one of my favourites. I ended up here by googling places six hours from England. I booked myself and three careers to go in November 2015, not really knowing what to expect. Well, after a very eventful flight, including a man who had a heart attack and a toddler playing boo over our chair for six hours straight, we arrived. Woowwwwww, the heat, and the manic-ness hit us right away. Here we soon learnt there were no rules; we could do anything, no health or safety. Paradise! I was lifted into a bus, wheelchair on the roof and we were off, avoiding cows on the motorway. There were people everywhere, lots just sitting enjoying the sun. We soon arrived at our gorgeous hotel on the beach and within hours we had gotten to know the hotel staff and had found our tour guide. We booked to see monkeys and crocodiles for our first outing.

On the day, a pickup arrived and I was lifted into the back; nothing was any trouble. The monkeys in the forest were amazing, coming right up to us, even fighting. Next, we saw the crocodiles at the sacred lake. Next day we got up and out early for a full day trip. Our truck for the day was a monster truck with ladders. Was it a problem? Nope, the tour guide lifted me onto his back and took me to his seat.

I was by this point being referred to as the 'empress'! During our day, we visited schools where they all sang to us, had lunch on a beach, visited a natural textile shop and a 'compound' which was very remote; it was where a lot of the locals would live. The lady allowed us to look around. I was so taken aback by their traditions; her son had married so he and his wife had an amazing room with a huge bed, while his Mum (the head of the house) slept on a mattress on the floor. Everywhere we went on our trip, children would run behind our truck. We were allowed to give out sweets – they literally had nothing.

Back at our hotel, we met some amazing people. There was a lifeguard, Midnight, who would do anything for me, helping me in and out of the water and taking me anywhere I wanted of a night. We were invited to the locals' bar; it was crazy, they had parties on the beach all night with homemade gin, but they looked after us and treated us as one of them.

During our week we did so much, never stopping. We visited markets and shops and one day went to a local orphanage. Imagine me - who isn't really child orientated – wanting to bring them all home. We had taken donations of books, crayons and clothes. They were so grateful, they lived at the orphanage until they were 18, even going to school there. The children's carers were amazing, treating them as their own. I could have stayed all day. The children loved my chair and were mesmerised by it and kept sitting on my knee. Another day, I felt I wanted to help more, so the tour guide, Yousef, took us to a goat farm where I bought two goats and took them with some rice to a local family. They were so grateful. The man of the family lived with his wife and children in a house made of corrugated iron with no flooring. When we gave him the goats, he said a prayer for us. I felt it was the least I could do and it wasn't much money to me, compared to the difference it would make to his family.

There was an endless list of things we could do. We went to a museum and were shown how the locals made their produce and we were shown how to play Gambian instruments.

The hotel put on different entertainment each night. We watched local African dancers and had chance to join in. One night the hotel had a power cut, so we all sat for ages in the pitch black. It was the best adventure – not bad for someone in a wheelchair. People thought I was crazy, heading to the middle of Africa, but I would go again any time. I was sad to be leaving this crazy, unusual but totally amazing place. I felt I could have filled at least another week but it was time to return home and I left with so many incredible memories.

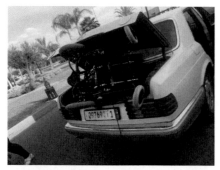

Morocco – May 2016

In May 2016, I went to Morocco. It was only four hours on a plane so I figured it would be OK… I was wrong. Getting on the plane was fine but at the other end I was taken off on the small airport wheelchair that is so unsuitable for me, so once off the plane I fell off it, landing on the floor. I was so angry and upset, not a great start to my holiday. Why is it so bloody hard not to drop me?? You would think being in this day and age that such a large and reputable airline company would have adequate means to get each and every one of their guests, on and off the aircraft safely and respectfully, this should be a basic right.

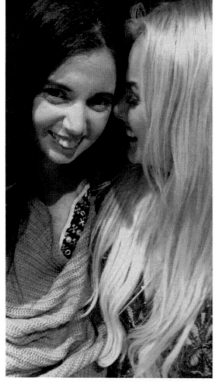

Morocco itself was amazing, so hot. I went on this holiday with my Mum, sister Sophie and friend Tom and three carers, so it was amazing to have some family time. We relaxed by the pool, went out to the Moon Bar in the town centre, which had stunning views, and we headed to the souks: the local markets. The markets were like a maze, with the most amazing clothes you could imagine. I learnt to haggle here; it's the only way to buy anything. You barter between you on a price. The atmosphere was amazing with the music and local people. I avoided the snake charmers but held monkeys and found a little basket with tortoises in one stall. Odd but cute. Everyone was very friendly but mostly they were intrigued by my chair.

One day we went to visit camels. I wasn't sure I would get on them, but the two guides made it easy, lowering the camel to a

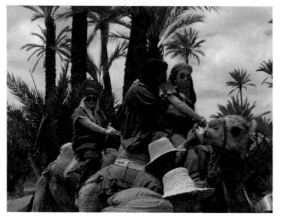

kneeling position and on I went with Tom. We all headed off, with my Mum's camel being naughty, biting all the other camels. The whole experience was incredible and we were all dressed up in robes with headwear. One more ticked off the bucket list!

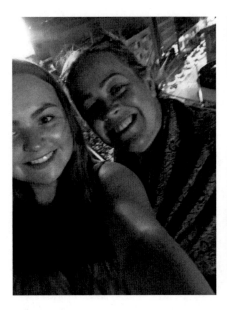 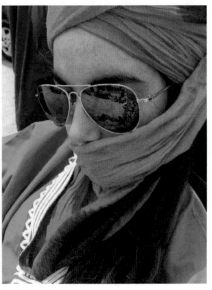 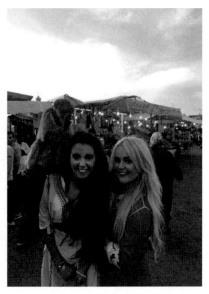

Next was a mud buggy safari, through the sand dunes on the edge of the desert. I was in a buggy with Karen, who was driving, and we followed our guide, who went really slowly. After a while we lost him and Karen put her foot down, speeding up and down the dunes with the wind in our hair, and arriving at the end covered head to toe in mud. Nothing's ever boring!

Our hotel was huge and wonderful. The only problem was that I found my bed so uncomfortable. By the end of our stay, we had borrowed sun loungers and mattresses, so I looked like princess and the pea.

On the last day, I was dreading the journey home and sure enough, it was bad. Everyone else was boarded onto the plane before me and then when I went on I was dropped in the aisle, (for the third time), and put in the wrong seat and had air conditioning dripping on my head all the way home. I was so angry and upset. I deserve to be treated with respect like everyone else. On landing in Manchester, the airline staff refused to help (aghhh!) so my carers physically carried me off. It was

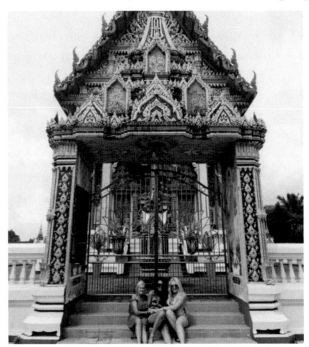

humiliating and a pity that after such an amazing experience away, this tainted it all. As you can imagine, a huge complaint went in to the airline.

Thailand – October 2017

In October 2017, I decided to really push myself and do the longest and furthest away place, my dream…. Thailand. It was a quite a journey…

We set off in the early hours in the morning; me, Mum and sister Sophie and my carer Karen, her partner Chris and teenage daughters, Erin and Niamh. Our first stage was a six and a half-hour flight to Saudi Arabia, followed by a four-hour stop over, then an eight-hour flight to Bangkok. Wow.

I can't say it was easy, but we managed it and all still smiling!

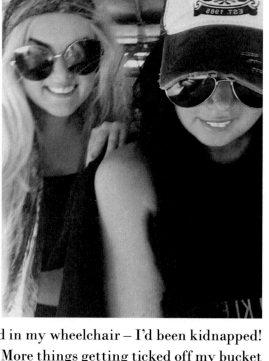

Bangkok was everything I imagined; a proper mega-city. We were met at the airport by Sombat, who was going to be our taxi driver for our time there. He was such a nice man. We headed straight to our hotel to get ready and unpack. Then off we went to explore. We were there the week of the king's funeral, so everywhere around Thailand there were portraits of him and yellow flowers. That night, we went to a huge shopping centre and ate by the harbour. The views were out of this world!

The next day was packed. We headed to an animal park, where we held baby tigers and orangoutangs. At one point the orangutang jumped down and started pushing me around in my wheelchair – I'd been kidnapped! He was so clever and so gentle. More things getting ticked off my bucket list! Next, we headed to the Koh San Road - the crazy part of Thailand. It's only one road, but anything goes! We met so many people and ate traditional Thai street food, including scorpions that come dried on a stick. They were vile; just all shell. After that we headed back to the hotel to change then to the tallest building in Bangkok, The Sky Bar, which has got the most insane views. There's even a clear platform where diners eat; it's totally made out of glass and juts out of the side of the building. Bangkok looked stunning of a night, it was worth the £26 we paid for one drink! Hahaha! Next Sombat took us on a tour and we saw lots of the temples and the grand palace, which was stunning but unfortunately, we couldn't go in, due to preparations for the funeral. Just seeing it was enough. We headed back to the hotel and had to be up early for our flight to Krabi. I was sad to be leaving Bangkok. I could have done with a few more days there.

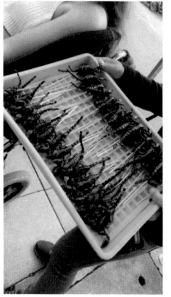

We left from Bangkok airport, which is smaller than the one we had flown into. The journey was so stressful, but it ended up being like something out of a film. We were late for the plane so were running through the airport then... we came to escalators. There were no lifts. Okkayyyy... I was stuck, but just as a feeling of dread hit us and we were thinking we would miss the flight, Chris decided to accept the challenge to get me down. He bounced my chair down the first flight of stairs than another set faced us – arghh! This time Chris got me on an escalator and we made it, to a noisy reception from our whole group, who were cheering. It could only happen to us.

After a pleasant flight, we arrived in Krabi .... Wowwwww what a contrast. There was greenery everywhere and no high-rise buildings; I loved it! Our hotel was gorgeous, both the place and the people. We were told that we had missed the monsoons by a few days, which was so lucky. All we did was change and chill by the pool. After the craziness of Bangkok, this was a totally different pace. I had massages and relaxed.

On exploring, not far from our hotel was the beach and a strip of shops and bars, which we spent many nights in. This is where my sister got pulled up on the stage to sing. Everybody was so friendly and laid back, nothing was too much trouble. My main goal was to visit the Phi Phi islands, so we found a tour guide and bartered a price. The next day we were off! We thought the islands wouldn't be far but an hour later we were still bouncing around in the speed boat! It was worth it; we first visited a cove that had the bluest water. It was so hot and lots of people were swimming. Next, we went to monkey island, where tourists threw food, and tiny monkeys dived into the water and swam to get the food... so cute!! Next, we visited Phi Phi Don - the main island. the sand was white and it was so hot, also very busy with so many tourists. There were shopping places, hotels and restaurants, so we spent time exploring then headed back to the boat. On the way back, we found a small cove and I got off the boat to snorkel. I never thought I could do it, but I tried and I did! I

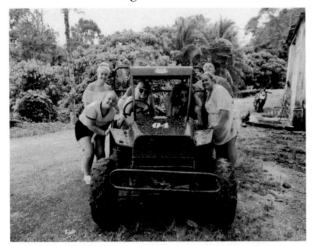

couldn't believe how far I'd come; how I was in the ocean snorkelling thousands of miles from home. This was a huge, huge high point! We headed home on the craziest boat ride; the tides were stronger and it was so bumpy. We got off wetter than if we'd been in the sea itself!

Whilst in Thailand, I had travelled on tuk tuks, buses, 4 x 4s and disco tuk tuks – so different from England, where I can't travel unless my chair is clipped in.

For the rest of our stay, we spent the days by the pool and of a night we visited local markets and got to know a massage shop over the road from our hotel, where daily they would spoil us with amazing treatments that were sooo cheap. When the day came to go, we were all so sad. We all just loved Krabi. We had the best last day on mud buggies, getting covered in mud and speeding round an off-road course, even having a couple of crashes. I loved every minute!

Our taxi took two hours to Phuket. Phuket was different again - somewhere in between Bangkok and Krabi. Our hotel was huge and right off the beach with a massive pool. Unlike Krabi, we

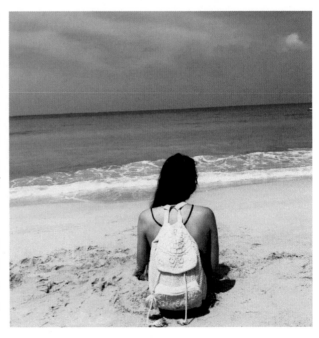

couldn't just walk around, but we met a lovely taxi driver who drove us every day. We visited Patong beach and we were caught in a tropical storm. We did lots of shopping and went to watch a fire walk. We also visited an orphanage that had been built after the tsunami, which had left lots of children homeless and without parents. I found this experience very emotional and it made me appreciate my family and everything I have even more.

The day of the king's funeral everywhere was shut and all staff wore black. There was a no-alcohol policy too out of respect. We decided to chill by the pool but we were soon horrified as a little boy fell into the pool and nearly drowned. Fortunately, after receiving care he was fine and the next day he was back like nothing had happened.

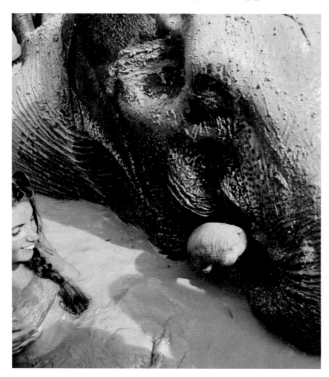

The highlight of my trip was a visit to the elephant retirement sanctuary. It is home to elephants that had been rescued from circuses or tourist places and they are now able to live a life where they could do as they please. We prepared food for them, fed them and spent lots of time with them. I found it out of this world. I was able to join in giving the elephants a mud bath, soon getting covered and then we went in a clear pool with them to wash off. I will remember this experience for the rest of my life.

As the holiday came to a close, I could only feel so grateful and proud of everything I had achieved. There is no stopping me: on to my next adventure. After that, I knew I could achieve anything. Now for the 15-hour flight home.

CHAPTER 8

Charity Work

I am blessed that I have so much support since my stroke. My life would be a shadow of what it is currently, without the support I receive. Sometimes thank you just doesn't seem enough, so I thought I'd show my gratitude in a more pro-active way.

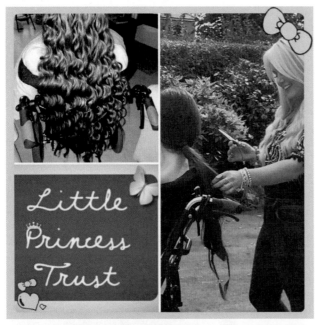

The Little Princess Trust – September 2015

Have you seen my hair? It's very long, so when I heard about the fantastic Little Princess Trust, which uses donated hair to make wigs for children who've been affected by cancer, I just knew straight away I wanted to help. My friends organised a tea party and raised such a lot of money for the cause, after I had inches cut from my tresses. Anyone who knows me, knows my hair is my pride and joy so this was quite an ordeal but well worth it.

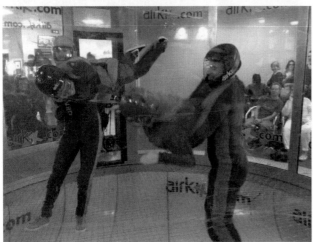

Indoor Skydive for Breast Cancer Research – September 2014

My brother's girlfriend is called Kelly; she's beautiful inside and out and I have a lot to do with her. One day she introduced me to her best friend, Di, who had breast cancer and the first time I met her I just knew I wanted to do something on her behalf. I was wracking my brain as to how I could help because I am obviously limited in what I can do. Eventually I decided to do a sky dive but no companies would accept me with their company. I didn't give up and later I heard about indoor skydiving in Manchester, so I set up a Just Giving page and started fundraising for Breast Cancer UK. My friend Amy and I did the indoor sky dive together. Not only was it fun but for those four minutes I felt free and light and it was so good not to have this ridiculous wheelchair attached to my bum! I'm so happy to say that I will be doing a real skydive with another friend later this year.

Orphanage fundraising - October 2015

During my travels in Gambia, we visited a local orphanage and were lifted by the happiness and spirit of the children. I actually got to Africa in the first place because my two best friends, Liv and Kate, did a fundraising event called "Get Mia to Africa" and that paid for me to go. We caused quite a commotion, turning up with my wheelchair, as I don't suppose they seen them very often. I took lots of books, pencils and pens with me to hand into the school and I donated money to them, which they used to assist more children to receive an education. A young Gambian boy, the son of one of the local men that had helped me while I was there, was having to travel for miles to get to school as his family couldn't afford the local school fees. I was glad I could fundraise to help with the fees. Within a week of getting home, I had set up a Just Giving page to get money together to fund him to go to school and for his uniform and books and pens. The whole trip was based around charity work, so all my spending money went to local people we met and was donated to various schools and orphanages. I was lucky enough to visit another orphanage while in Thailand, again a bright and happy place. My family don't send Christmas cards each year now, but instead donate to this orphanage.

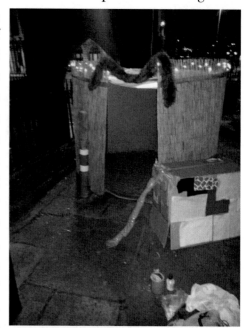

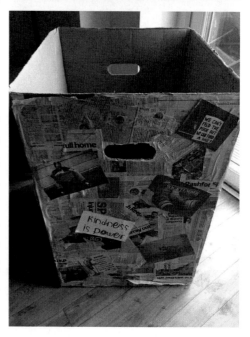

Helping the Homeless

In October 2014, I began collecting old winter clothing to donate to the Whitechapel Centre in Liverpool, which gives invaluable support to homeless people in the city. Donating unwanted coats, hats, scarves and gloves gives the charity a little boost. I didn't feel this was enough though, so to really get an understanding of how it feels to be homeless, I spent a night in the churchyard in the 'Liverpool Sleep-out'. We made a makeshift shelter and had thermals and a sleeping bag but I still felt bitterly cold, so how must someone feel night after night?

Calais – October 2016

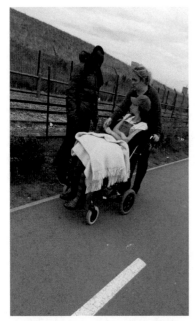

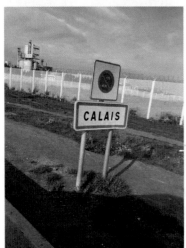

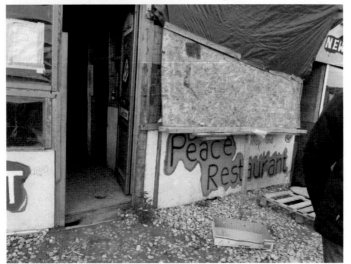

The cold was also something I considered when I thought about the refugees stranded at Calais. With fast winter quickly approaching, I knew I just had to help. It was October 2016 and I had been watching on the TV for a while about the situation in Calais, so I decided to set up my own appeal. Over several weeks I collected lots of donations, especially clothes. Not only that but I felt I wanted to travel to Calais by ferry to give the refugees the donations face to face. With my car loaded to the brim with clothes, shoes and blankets, Karen, Jess and I spent three days travelling to 'the Jungle' and back, to hand out all the winter essentials that had kindly been donated. I was shocked to my core at what I saw and the conditions people were living in.

It was deeply harrowing experience and so dangerous in fact that an hour after my departure the embassy stopped all ferries to France, as there was a huge political debate going on. I filled my car to the brim and set off with my carers, Karen and Jess. After 7 hours driving, we arrived at the ferry, after a few hours on the ferry we arrived in Calais. We witnessed the devastation as soon as we arrived. There were huge camps at the side of the road as we drove towards the town, but we were blocked by police. Instead we went down the main road next to the camp, which was also full of refugees. We set to work straight away giving out donations. They were desperate for clothes and especially gloves. I met a variety of people among the refugees during my time there and they would sit and tell me their stories. They were very highly intelligent and from various different countries. They were all so polite and friendly. Whereas the propaganda tells us the Jungle is a violent place to be, in fact it was the police in France that were violent: they beat the refugees and shot rubber bullets at the children. It was soul destroying.

We gave so much out. I even gave out my turkey batches, that were my food for the day. The refugees explained that they sat in the streets because conditions in the actual camp were so bad. We felt we needed to help more so headed back to our hostel, where we just booked a basic room that we could just about fit into. It wouldn't feel right booking anything more. The next day we set out early and headed straight to

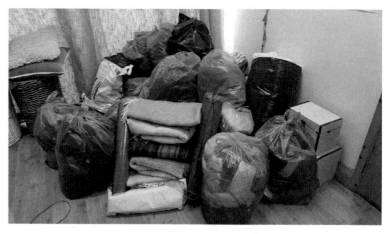

the road by the camp, finding it full of police who were trying to close the camp down. The poor refugees were getting hit and sworn at. It was so upsetting. We weren't allowed to stop, so did what we could and went back later with phone credits that we bought. We got out and gave the credits to the men who we had got to know. Next minute I saw someone looking over a shoulder trying to pinch someone else's number. This made me really mad, until Karen noticed and got Jess to cover the number. I met a guy from Sudan who was a doctor and he took my wheelchair where the news broadcasters were desperately warning people not to go – into the actual Jungle. Before we came we had decided we wouldn't venture in, as we didn't think it was safe, but with them showing us we decided to go in for a few minutes. It was out of this world, the way the poor people were living. I went white. I wasn't scared at all but reality hit me: every inch was tent after tent and this is what the refugees had to face every day. Remarkably they weren't all sad; and the atmosphere was lovely. We were just glad to have been able to help in a small way.

Socktember 2017

Not everything is doom and gloom and there are really some fun ways to raise money to help others. Take for instance the Splash Dash at Aintree racecourse in aid of breast cancer research; well, let's just say that the dye gets everywhere! Ha ha ha! Getting everyone to donate their old and new socks for the needy is also fun. I collected lots of socks to help the homeless and took them to a homeless shelter in Liverpool. 361 pairs were a big help for Socktember!

Parking

Fortunately, 95% of my neighbours are absolutely fantastic, lovely people but there's always a few who aren't. We had a nightmare with parking, for example; one couple left three threatening notes for my personal assistant so I demanded to go up to these neighbours and he was horrible to me and said, 'It's not my fault what happened to you but it's an inconvenience.' Another neighbour barged into my house uninvited shouting about parking in the vicinity of her house so when my sister went round for a word about resolving this matter the woman put her hand in my sister's face and said just shut up will you. If people park near your house in the future, please take a minute to empathise with the reason why. I hope these neighbours don't need carers in the future because there are no bus stops nearby.

A Glass Half Empty or Half Full? Obviously Overflowing!

I never believed in the half full —
half empty bullshit, what I always knew was that some of us had something in the glass and some of us didn't and I've always been willing to pour mine out so that others could have something rather than nothing.

– Joe Straynge.

I hear people explain my situation sometimes and the other person inevitably responds sympathetically, 'Awww!' But it's not aww really 70% of the time because I made the decision to wake up and suck it up and I'm still standing by this. Though it does really annoy me when people moan, especially on days that I feel rubbish about what has happened but I don't say anything. I know everyone is entitled to have a moan every now and then but in the grand scheme of things I find people don't realise how lucky they are and often take the little things in life for granted.

Ambitions

You might wonder whether my ambitions are anything like those you'd expect of someone who is approaching 30 years of age and with a lively character. From my perspective, most people's aim in life is to have a mortgage and a family, whereas I just want genuine happiness and to travel with my sister. Though my real ambition is to become a worldwide investigator like Reggie Yates and Stacey Dooley, with my sister as my voice.

Doctors and Follow-ups

Follow up appointment? What follow up appointment? I left hospital with one physio appointment where they taught the agency carers a range of stretching exercises, which the carers never did once and I was told I didn't meet the health service requirements for physio… SERIOUSLY?

I totally understand the politics and the mess we are in when it comes to health care so instead of getting angry I have been doing my own physio and hydro and even organised a rehabilitation period where I booked myself into a local hotel with a gym and a pool.

I devised a rehabilitation plan for myself, which consisted of gym, swim, salt therapy and oxygen therapy. My rota was so strict and every day I had something on and it started to really help but then I got a chest infection and was advised not to swim or do oxygen therapy or do the physio so I had to come home. Luckily, the hotel were great about it. I had begun to slowly improve but when the chest infection started it was game over and I felt a bit defeated. I'd definitely do anything like this again, but there are very limited places that provide this and it was either £9000 or flying abroad for treatment.

Oxygen Therapy

I began going to oxygen therapy sessions. Each session involves 1.5 hours in a hyperbaric chamber and I came back totally enlightened. I should – and did – get oxygen treatment on a weekly basis but I had to stop this therapy because the oxygen was making me cough more. I remember being there one day and having to stop and disconnect from the oxygen because I was in floods of tears due to the pressure hurting my ears. A lady said she was in for cancer treatment and had been given 12 months to live. I suddenly felt it was so selfish to cry in front of her and spelt out, 'Sorry for reacting the way I did.' She really inspired me though as even with such a terrible prognosis she still has the strength to sort out therapies to prolong her life just a little bit more. When you put situations like this into perspective, it really angers me that vain, pretentious people use up oxygen therapy places purely for cosmetic reasons.

From my diary: *I had my second dose of oxygen therapy yesterday. I feel awful for saying that I feel a big difference because yesterday I met a gorgeous little four-year-old Chinese girl, also called Mia. She was coming for oxygen therapy every day with her condition, which I think is cerebral palsy. It's crazy how that little girl will never know how much of a difference she has made to me but she was such a cute, happy girl getting on with it and watching Peppa Pig on her iPad. It makes me think I should just shut up and get on with it myself! At least I will get back to normal eventually but her condition will never go, it'll just improve. It is going to take some getting used to for me to go because for the last six years I have avoided situations where I meet people with daily stresses, as opposed to surrounding myself with just family and friends. It's so sad when everyone is sat around waiting for the oxygen chamber to be ready and discussing why they are there. It breaks my heart to see kids whose parents are clearly trying literally every option to help. One lady yesterday said she had come over from Switzerland with her grandkids just for the oxygen therapy for three weeks.*

My eyes still fill up now thinking about all these children; how can I ever feel sad when I'm surrounded by inspirational children and adults defying the odds.

Back to the NHS

Anyway six years passed and I have to say I didn't hear a thing from the NHS so I had to demand an appointment with the consultant. It was about getting botoxin injections to ease the pain and spasm I get in my legs. I have botox in my legs regularly, done by my consultant, and I would love to say it works but without physio to maintain it, it seems pointless. I don't know why I go back – it is soul destroying. I totally understand that the doctors can give you false hope but it wouldn't harm them to say, 'The botoxin is not working but you're doing fantastic with your own progress and in everything you do.' Now I'm insecure about how ill I really am and have no confidence that my physio can improve and that I can go out and join in. Unfortunately, this is a huge downside to being ill, as is how dreadful my immune system is. It is so important to keep healthy, to avoid germs (not easy when I have so many people around me every day) and make sure my nutrition is good, so that I don't fall victim to the dreaded chest infections or, worse still, pneumonia – that really does stop me going out to play.

Opinions

Everyone is entitled to an opinion, especially those with direct encounters with the NHS for such a long length of time so here goes...

The doctors and registrars/ general practitioners and surgical nurses have been fantastic and really helpful and I've been seeing them for eight years on and off. However, the experience I've had with some nurses has been dreadful. Fortunately, I'm switched on enough not to let these disgusting human beings tarnish the reputation of the health service, because they are ultimately here for me although it's hard to forget the misery these people have caused. I just cling to the belief that karma is a bitch. It's a shame though, because for every bad nurse there's a multitude of fantastic, dedicated and brilliant ones. Another huge plus to the service has been my personal health budget, which allows me to fund Mia's Angels, my carers, and the various therapies, including the physio with Mark.

CHAPTER 9

Bucket List

Then it hit me one day... to write a bucket list. It consisted of just the sort of things that young people my age include in their adventures. And slowly I began to plan my first thing to do; a 30mph zip-line ride across Snowdonia with my sister Sophie.

The bucket list also included various things to be done abroad but it also said, 'make a difference', which I've hopefully done. I did a fundraiser event myself for the neurology ward, as well as a second indoor skydive in aid of cancer research and I cut off nine inches of my hair to raise money for the Little Princess Trust, to make a wig for a child who had lost their hair through illness or due to receiving cancer treatment. Often, I would take a donation to the homeless centre and I did the Liverpool Sleep-Out event but no one was prepared for the lengths I would go to help people.

My Bucket List

For the record, here's my bucket list. If you've been paying attention, you'll see that I've crossed some of them off already – just a few more to go!

Go on a motorbike
Stand between two borders
Go to London to see my cousins
Go to Bounce Below
Go to Iceland to the pool
Go to Finland and Norway
Meet Olly Murs and Will Young
Go to Jamaica
Do a skydive
Do a paraglide
Go to Scotland and Ireland for night out
Go to a crime scene
Work with Stacey Dooley and Reggie Yates
Dye my hair
Go to V Festival and Glastonbury

Climb Snowdon
Go to the jungle
Meet a tribe in the Amazon rainforest
Go to Ethiopia
Foster a child from Chernobyl
Volunteer in a soup kitchen
Be in a TV studio audience
Wingsuit flight
Free dive in the Bahamas
Great Barrier Reef dive
Dog sledding
Cage of death (Australia)
Chill factor

Zipwire – March 2014

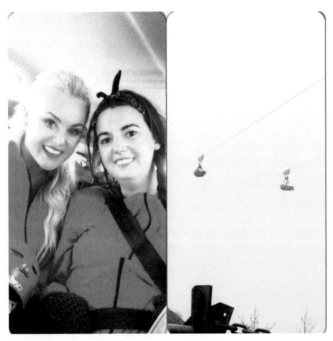

In March 2014, I decided to go to the zipwire in Snowdonia; it's the country's longest zipwire. I asked if it was suitable for me to do and straight away they said, 'Yes!' On arrival, I was given a jumpsuit, and then a Land Rover pulled up to take me to the start, but at that time I wasn't able to stand as well as I can now, so we were worried it was going to be cancelled. With sheer determination, we gave it a go and I was able to get into the Land Rover to go up the hill, taking the wheelchair on the back. Then we hit a flight of stairs arghh! but nothing stops me. So I was carried up and put in the harness. It took about twenty minutes to fasten me but it was worth it! Poor Sophie was doing the zipwire with me and got left to sort herself out, while everyone fussed over me lol. My Mum and Dad were absolute wrecks but I was determined to cross a zip-wire ride off my bucket list. I was all hooked up in my red boiler suit thinking, 'Shit! What was I thinking?' But I couldn't back out now because I had about twenty people fussing over me and next thing I knew it was 3..2..1.. SHITTT! I was going. It felt like I was flying, it was amazing but I honestly did feel as though my head was going to fall off. I closed my eyes the whole distance until just before the end, looking across to my sister, who was adjacent with wide eyes as if to say, 'NEVER AGAIN!' My Mum and Dad were there at the bottom. I honestly can't believe I did it. From being in the hospital, unable to move more than my eyes, to flying over mountains feeling totally free was surreal. But after I came home pumped with adrenaline, I booked my next activity, which was a mud buggy and sure enough I did that and then went on to book my shark dive, and then my indoor skydive and then the indoor skiing, zorbing, bungee – and so it carried on.

I have the bug now; I'm a complete adventure junkie.

Shark Dive – February 2015

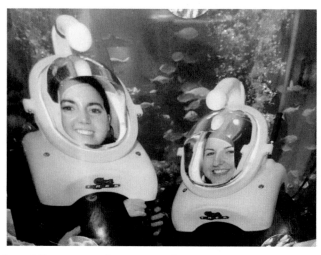

In February 2015, I completed a shark dive. I had wanted to do it for so long but because the stroke made it difficult to coordinate my breathing, I knew I would be unable to scuba dive and use the breathing equipment correctly. Then I discovered in the Sea Life Centre in Trafford Park, where they use oxygen-filled helmets. We spoke to them and after lots of discussion, I was booked to do it. I arrived with family and lots of friends, ready to watch my friend Amy and I accept the challenge. After changing into our wetsuits, we discovered that the way up to the tank is via stairs – and lots of them! It was at this point that my carer's partner just picked me up over his shoulder and give me a fireman's lift to the top.

They gave me the helmet and put me into the water. I couldn't see what was below me at that point, as I was told not to look down. If I had, my helmet would have filled with water. I was taught the divers' communication signals – and they were taught mine – then off I went. I was lowered in

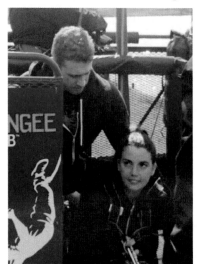

and I knew everyone was holding their breath, checking I was OK. In fact, I was fine; I could breathe as normal, the divers took me down and I was surrounded by huge sharks, fish and sea turtles. I absolutely loved it. The divers were amazing and helped me to walk all around the tank. I loved looking through the huge glass screen seeing everybody there. Another adventure ticked off my bucket list!

Bungee Jumping – 2015

In 2015, I decided to do a bungee jump. Even people that knew about my adrenaline streak thought I was crazy and everyone prayed the bungee people would say no but guess what? They said yes!

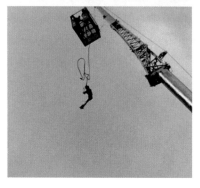

I went to Tatton Park in Manchester, where I was confronted by a crane, hundreds of feet in the air. This time my partner in crime was Mark, my personal trainer. On arrival, I got ready and my harness was attached. They were originally concerned that the rope might damage my neck on falling, but they managed to attach it somewhere elsewhere, to avoid that problem. They placed me inside the lift of the crane but as my legs decided not to cooperate, I was going higher and higher with the crane door open and my legs sticking out. My adrenaline was going crazy, we went so high. At the top, there was a count to three and I was falling, faster and faster. It was amazing! Then I was bounced back up; it was so scary but over so quickly and I immediately wanted to go again. While I waited to be lowered, I could just hear cheers and claps from everyone below. I came down to see my Mum's relieved face; she had thought the plan was that I was coming down tandem. She also pointed out the red rope mark on my face where the rope had slipped and hit me. I didn't even notice, I was too excited! It was incredible. Poor Mark was next. He was white going up and once at the top he remained still for over five minutes. I think he felt even more pressure, going after me, that he had to jump, but he was frozen. In the end, he was pushed off by the staff (he agreed, haha!), but once down, he vowed, 'Never again!', whereas I was already thinking of my next adventure.

One Love Festival – September 2015

2015 was turning into such a busy year. In the summer, I went to the One Love Festival. It was a reggae festival, the music I love! I went with my carer, Karen, and carer/friend Louin, who is very similar to myself. It was down south from where I live, so we went with a car-full of supplies and a tent. We got there and got set up quickly and out. First, I went zorbing on water with Lou. Thinking of getting me into the large, transparent globe of the zorb it seemed as though it would be difficult, but it was actually straightforward. There were so many people at the festival and lots of tents, where bands were playing different types of music. I positioned myself at the front of the tents and danced so much. (I can manage to dance with my sister or my friends around me to stop me from falling. I feel very involved because people are so sensitive and involve me.)

I enjoyed every second, and met such a variety of people; from the crazy blonde who thought she was the best dancer, but after a lot of drink it turned out that she wasn't, to the homeless vegan man, it was crazy. Lou was granting wishes for people by blowing fairy dust on them, and I on the other hand was getting attention from a man who kept offering me his mother's scarf. I was quite happy just dancing but then suddenly his girlfriend appeared, kicking off in my face! Lou and Karen tried to sit me back but I wasn't having it, I wouldn't sit back, I stood my ground. In the end, the man pulled her off and explained to her that it was him, not me, and she couldn't apologise enough.

At nights we were kept up by a group of girls in a tent next to us and so our last night, Lou invited people back to ours as payback! We spent our last day on the grass, listening to music under the sun with amazing people. Our little homeless man taught us a lot; he made the most of life and stuck to his beliefs of being a vegan. I spent my last money buying him food. We went home penniless, but it was worth it!

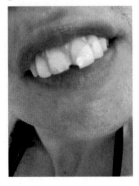

'Mia, don't panic, your teeth are in your hair!'

An exciting item still left on my bucket list was to go on a speedboat, so on a weekend away of May 2017, we went on a speedboat in Abersoch. It was fantastic but because of how I landed in the boat, my two front teeth came out...

Luckily, my friend Pip is a dental nurse and put me in touch with her friend Natalie who thankfully took me on and replaced my teeth with veneers. I now have the most perfect natural smile.

Gay Pride – August, annually

Every year I go to the Gay Pride festival in Manchester. It is always epic and has never let me down.

I go and meet my friends from Preston and always have the wildest time. This year I went with my sister Sophie, my cousins Liv and Kate, and friends Erin, Nic and Karen. Every year they have so much to do and it usually starts with the parade, which is so impressive. This year I went just for the nightlife.

The concert was massive. I got right to the front and I was enjoying the music when suddenly I noticed that two hen parties were having a physical fight right next to me. At one point my friends were thinking of putting me right over the barriers to keep me safe. We eventually managed to get away and left them to it. So many mad things have happened there. One year a guy I didn't know just decided to hold my hand throughout the concert. I love it because everything there is acceptable and everyone can just be themselves. It is the polar opposite of normal but that is why I love it!

One Tribe Festival – August 2017

For my birthday, I went with Sophie and our best friend Pip, to the 2017 One Tribe Festival in Cheshire. The atmosphere was incredible. The niche market was predominantly hippies and yes, they were more than likely stoned, but we loved it. They had a rave inside the forests and lots of tents, all with insane music. I love a festival and everything that goes with it. I look forward to them because they break up each year for me; they can be long otherwise!

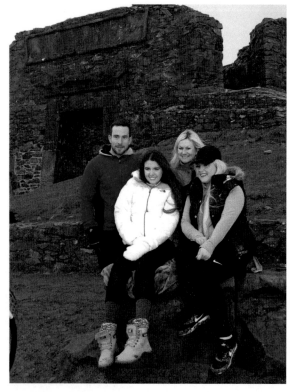

Moel Famau – January 2017

Without giving myself praise, I know that I have accomplished many things since my stroke. Last year I was given the most amazing present by my old friend, Rich. I know I've mentioned Rich before and how supportive he was when I had my stroke. We continued our relationship for about two years after the accident but unfortunately it was getting difficult to even see each other. I'd have back to back meetings and by 6pm I just had no energy and wanted time to breathe and rest my eyes. So it ended but we are still great friends and have still gone out and done the most incredible things together.

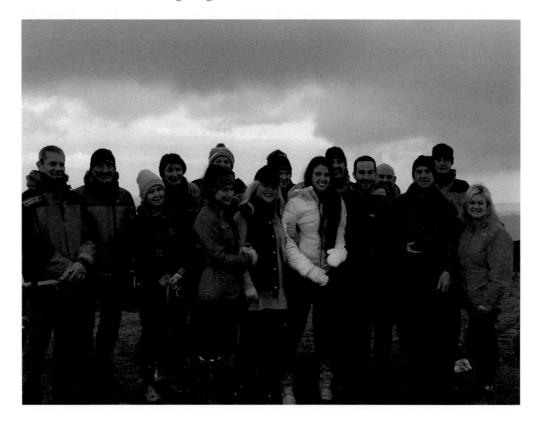

It had been my ambition to go to the top of Moel Famau with Rich once again, something I was told would not be possible after my stroke. The hill is the highest point for miles around and we'd previously climbed it together. Before the accident, this was our thing and we climbed it quite often. I was a very active person with much enthusiasm for the great outdoors. Rich had organised with the local mountain rescue team to assist me up to the top in a vehicle. It was a lovely bright but crisp and cool day when the team met me and many of my friends and family along with loads of volunteers and dogs. They treated me like a V.I.P., taking me up the mountain in a Land Rover, while the others walked. I was in my element at the top of Moel Famau, totally taken back and left breathless by the views of the surrounding towns. People assisted me to stand up so I could get good-quality photos with my beloved friends and family and the very much appreciated mountain rescue team. Then they helped me back into the Land Rover and we started our descent down the mountain. Even then the view going back down took my breath away; you could see hang-gliders passing by. I could not be more appreciative to the mountain rescue team and Rich himself for allowing me to live this dream once again. We gave a generous donation to the mountain rescue team and said our goodbyes, then we headed for some drinks to warm us up. This was one of the most amazing days.

CHAPTER 10

ATTITUDES

Intelligence

I strongly believe the less you speak the more intelligent you get and it's incredible the things you pick up on when you're not speaking and take time to listen.

Regrets

People ask me whether I regret anything but to be honest, I regret eating that whole chocolate orange from this morning's breakfast more, ha! Then again, do people really think I had had time to do stuff that I might regret now? I was only just getting into the swing of life.

Moaners

People moaning drives me absolutely mad. When they say, 'Aaww, I've ripped my nail!' I just stare at them and raise one eyebrow and think, 'Seriously?!'

Prankster

I'm the biggest prankster ever! For example, I always pretend to cough and choke and when people say, 'It's a shame!' I start to dribble and cross my eyes.

Stress

I often see the cool kids who were bullies toward me before my stroke and I hope they look at me and think, 'I added to the stress that caused that.' Not that I will ever know 100% the cause but I can't come to any other conclusion than that I was under severe stress.

Who are you looking at?

I find that people who are curious about me don't just slyly look at me but fully gawp for a substantial amount of time, which is funny to me because if only they could hear what I'm thinking about them! I have travelled to many different countries and, although you rarely see people in wheelchairs, there they are less likely to stare. Considering the UK is meant to be at the forefront of inclusion, it is much worse.

Disabled? Not me!

The only problem I've had since my stroke is that I simply won't and can't accept that I'm disabled. I have an issue with the word and wouldn't put myself in that bracket. I'm everything disabled is not. You think a disabled person is on average a vulnerable un-able, poorly-looked-after person in a home in any old clothes, smelling of piss with fish pie stains down their jumper, a tartan blanket, black eyes, pale skin, thick yellow nails and stuck in front of TV. I am the total, total opposite; I take pride in my appearance, I won't even eat in public but most of all I'm an absolute wild child.

Positivity

It's not negative that this happened to me when I was so young. In fact, it's so positive because I'm young enough to be retrained, whereas when you're old, the likelihood is that it will have a detrimental effect and you wouldn't really battle to get better at ninety.

Laughs – some funny things that keep my spirits up:

A carer slipped on decking so I bought her an anti-slip mat.

I sent a photo to a carer and coloured her eye in green, she was convinced I'd poked myself in the eye with a pen.

A carer once put conditioner on my legs instead of after-sun lotion.

I asked a carer to open a door as I was hot but she opened the wardrobe door.

When we were out in the car, we warned a carer she would hit a petrol pump and she said, 'Yes, I know,' but she drove forward and hit it anyway.

Then there was the day that my male carer dressed up in my clothes, pretending to be me.

Or my naughty dog, Dolly, stealing the carer's food.

Not to mention lots and lots of crazy nights out.

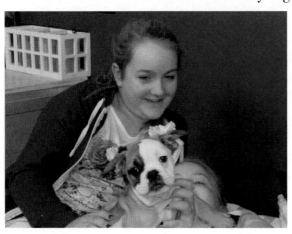

Dolly Austin

I got Dolly in 2014 as a puppy; she is a bulldog and is such a smart dog with such amazing character. She is so affectionate and is always so gentle with me. She's so funny as she bosses my carers around and when they come into my room to help me she comes too. She's the most amazing dog.

CHAPTER 11

Current Situation

Cough, cough

Recently, I've been getting lots of chest infections, one after the other. Even courses of antibiotics aren't helping, so I'm doing lots to build my immune system up. Taking vitamins, drinking lots of water, visiting a salt cave in Liverpool and I also have a salt machine in my room. This has really been especially helpful. It is completely natural but has so many benefits, so hopefully my chest infections won't come back.

My Subconscious

I find it amazing how differently I behave subconsciously. Since having the stroke, I have done many things without realising, like at night I full on bend my legs and put them out of the bed. I think I'm subconsciously trying to escape but some would call it a muscle spasm. It's amazing how countless times carers have come in of a night and found my legs off the bed when I'm asleep; it's almost as if my body is awake. My doctor's notes mention me sleep walking and when I say 'no' it comes out in a cockney accent, although I can't talk. Once I was sunbathing in the garden and I automatically pushed up my sunglasses when they fell down. In the beginning, I found it hard to shout for my carers but after years of shouting at them in my sleep, my voice got stronger. The subconscious mind baffles me.

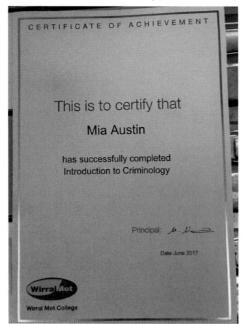

CERTIFICATE OF ACHIEVEMENT

This is to certify that

Mia Austin

has successfully completed
Introduction to Criminology

Principal:

Date June 2017

WirralMet
Wirral Met College

Seven-year cycle

Someone once told my Mum that the human brain regenerates itself every seven years. This is year seven and I'm pushing myself with different therapies to stimulate any sleeping parts.

College

My goal in life, regardless of what happened is to be treated equally and as no less. I do find that a lot of people treat me like I'm stupid but, in my view, they would be stupid to think that. Continuing my education not only integrates me to society but makes me a more informed about this new world around me. So far, I have done a criminology course at Conway Park in June 2017 and shortly after that, I took it upon myself to complete a forensics course online with the Open University. Starting in 2018, I will be undertaking another college course in criminal justice. Access to the college and the classroom is very easy, and tutors treat me like an equal. All I want is equality and opportunity. Although how everyone pulls themselves out of bed at half seven is beyond me!

Mobility

Do you know what? People expect me to have so many mobility issues with the new laws and regulations but my answer is SO WHAT if there are steps and doors that are not widened? I will always find a way to get around, whatever issues arise. Luckily for me, my family and friends and care team are incredible; they always find ways and wouldn't dream of making me feel inferior to what others can do. For example, in Morocco, we saw a camel excursion but not even an eyebrow was raised as to getting me on this seven-foot creature. Everyone just mucked in and got me on ensuring I got the full experience and that is how it should be viewed by everyone. I'd rather snap my neck bungee jumping and break every bone in my body than stay at home in my room, it is just a risk you take and without these people there would be no be no action Barbie! I am told life is for living so I intend to live the hell out of it!!!!

CHAPTER 12

—ᴡᴏᴄᴛᴏᴏᴛᴏᴏᴍ—

Living with it

Well, what can I say that is enough to make anyone understand, except emphasise

IT'S SHIT

But what can you do but adapt?

Don't get me wrong, some days I look in the mirror and repulsed by the new me and think, 'What the hell?'

But the lucky thing is your looks don't mean that much; they aren't important to anyone with a brain.

It is all about personality...

And I have a huge one of those!

Conclusion

To conclude my story, who knows what will happen physically, I'm only human, but I'm so grateful for everyone around me and I will continue to push myself. 'Life isn't about waiting for the storm to pass, it's about learning to dance in the rain.' I'll be forever happy no matter what; just me and my beautiful, amazing, kind, fluffy sister travelling the world together because, as our matching bracelets say, 'If no one understands, she does.'

In my life, all I have now is the desire to get up and travel the world, and I have this urge to help the school orphanages and poorer people. Although some sights rip my heart into a million pieces, ultimately it is just overwhelming and it makes me so happy to help and puts life into perspective.

I hope that I've persuaded people in similar positions that it's not all bad and only you can choose your destination in life. To their family and friends, just keep going and doing what you're doing because even one smile changes everything.

Poems to keep me going:

Fairies, Rainbows and Butterflies

Don't judge me because I'm in a chair
Because it's certainly not all rainbows and butterflies over there

I dribble sometimes because I can't swallow my spit
And my legs shoot out when they see fit
Sometimes I laugh but I mean to cry
I determine what I say using my eyes
I have OCD; I'm like a fairy with broken wings
And sit there and spot these little things
I look a mess sometimes because I can't do it all myself
I try and try again because I won't ask for help
All these things are a real pain
But my goal is to be seen the same!

A Pocket Full of Dreams

In my jeans is a pocket full of dreams
Including a time machine
I rewind back three years
No more frustration, no more tears
I'd do all the things I want to achieve
I'd say all the things I believe
I'd skydive from the highest height
And ask Mike Tyson for a fight
I'd travel round the world and back
With just my sunglasses and rucksack
I'd have a dance off with Diversity
And have a go at being an M.C.
I'd roll around in a chocolate bath
And get my friends round for a laugh
I'd drink champagne and go on a yacht
I'd get a pet monkey and call it Dot
I'd go and save kids all over the world
And feed and play with the little boys and girls.
I'd fly to space and step on the moon
This is all my dream but I'll be back soon!
Life is for living so do everything now
You never know when your time is up and you will get knocked down

abc easy as 1, 2, 3?

For one minute don't tell me it's easy to do
It's not as simple as teaching me animal names around the zoo
Will everyone stop telling me what I should do,
I'd give me a break, if I were you!

It's far from lying in bed and watching daybreak
So shut up and give me a rest, for goodness' sake.

Take a Picture, It Will Last Longer!

Why the hell do people feel the need to stop and stare at me?
It might be unusual to be in a chair at 23,
But what gives you the right to stare?
I'm a human with feelings under there!
Didn't your parents teach you it's rude to stare?
Big deal. I'm a normal girl with brown hair.
I'm locked up at the mo, but need the key,
Hey, you don't get away with staring at me!!

Mirror, mirror

I want a thinner nose
I want bigger boobs
I wish I could get away with wearing high shoes
I wish I had a nice flat belly
And my thighs didn't look like jelly
I want collar bones like Kendal Jenner
And hair like the girls from Wella
But it's 2016 and anything goes
We should all just appreciate that we have fingers and toes
Who really wants to be the girl on TV who makes herself sick
And is in massive financial deficit?
They even admit their real life ain't great
And when they look in the mirror they still feel hate.

Rule-breaker

I'm ready to stand up and act like a clown
But the doctors and physio moan, 'It's safe to sit down.'
Luckily I don't listen to my rulers
Because now I do everything sooner!
They are obsessed with doing everything right
They aren't used to people who put up a fight
Personally I think the rules are full of shite
At the end of the day I'm in one piece
So important people stop trying to give me grief!

In a Cage

It started by falling on the bathroom floor,
And followed with the sound of an ambulance door.
I woke from the coma, surrounded by machines,
All I can remember was having weird dreams.
The operation to be fed was the scariest of all,
Even worse than not being able to walk, talk or call.
Each day I was passed from pillar to post,
No-one cared what I needed the most.
Shoved in a wheelchair I had to grin and bear,
Left to sit alone, to think and stare.
I celebrated Christmas in a hospital room,
And by summer I was eating from a spoon.
The moral of my story is when people say
'Live each day as if it is your last'
Don't mope around, just go for it and have a blast!

Frustration

Sometimes I want to stomp and shout!
Why does no-one get what having a stroke is all about?
Why do people argue about funding my care?
And why is finding nice carers so rare?
Why can't everyone just read my mind?
Instead of spelling letters out all the time?
Why does everything take months on end?
And why does the NHS drive me around the bend?
Why do people talk to me in sign?
And most important…
Why do I bother getting wound up all the time?

Food

I dream about eating all sorts of food,
Like the biggest chocolate fountain in the world.
Spaghetti Bolognese, McDonalds, crisps, chicken and chips, strawberry laces, Nutella, calzone,
    garlic bread, carrots and chips.
Yogurts, Chewits, Refresher bars, Nancy's jacket potatoes, Domino's, Marmite, bread with balsamic
    dip, cucumber, cereal, cheese, Doritos.
Pick-and-mix, toast, crackers, bread sticks, rosemary potatoes, chocolate bars, fudge cake, hot
    chocolate…..

I wish I could eat even just one of those things.
I wasn't to know what life would bring.

Home, Sweet Home

Home, sweet home, where I belong
I can play music as loud as I like
Without next door putting up a fight
The clinical smell of hospital care
Has been replaced by Seabank Road sea air.
Although it was so hard to leave
Everyone around me is so pleased
To see Miss Austin gallivanting up and down her road
Even when the weather's freezing cold.
Back to safety and family fights,
But home, sweet home... feels so right.

Appreciation

Appreciate walking
Appreciate talking
Appreciate laughing
Appreciate freedom
Appreciate eating
Appreciate drinking
Appreciate sitting
Appreciate singing
Appreciate people
Appreciate shopping
Appreciate memories
Appreciate moving
Appreciate family
Appreciate everything
Be grateful for all you do
Because even if it seems tiny, it's HUGE to me.

Adventure

Who thought I'd be travelling forty hours from my bed
When just a few years ago I was off my head.
From plane to plane, travelling again,
Around the world, no day is the same.

Challenging yourself is a good place to start,

Gathering your courage and following your heart.

So save all your pennies, and exchange into baht.

In life people want babies, puppies and a nice cosy home,

But all I want to do is wonder and roam.

What is life without adventure and risk,

Don't hold back: life is too brisk.

CHAPTER 13

THANKS

To Debbie

I have a ginormous sense of appreciation for a lady called Debbie who, despite all the issues I've had with NHS, has totally restored my faith in the service. She manages all my funding I get to pay for all my carers and has opened my eyes to the fact that they are there to help and they are on my side. I don't know where I'd be without this help and her utter dedication. After being told the service could not fund my physio for years she straightaway built this into my budget and gave the go-ahead for me to get the cough machine I so very much needed. So, although the service has their baddies, they also have some saints. Without doubt, the majority are brilliant and say they get far too much negative press. The passion Debbie has about the patients in her care inspires me to want to be like her and fight for a service we all rely on at some stage.

To Mark

Thanks Mark, you didn't train me to do a marathon, nor did you train me to look good, but you trained me to save my life. You made me move, you made me eat well and ultimately made me believe in myself again.

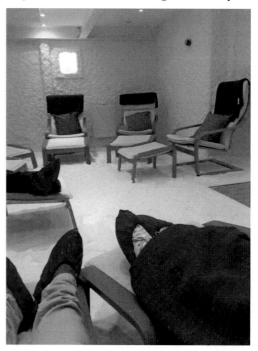

To Mia's Angels

I would like to say thank you to all my Angels. You will never know just how special you are and you have played a huge part in my life.

To my Friends

Because of my friends I cry less and smile more. Many thanks also to my friends; Mike, Ben, Siân, Amy, Pip, Saffron, Kelly, Chris, Nic, Liv and Kate, Amy for standing by me when I've needed friends the most. Thank you to

Rob and Rich and every one that fundraises for me because it is you that paid for me to get home get settled and to lead the life I have now.

To the Salt Cave, Liverpool

Thank you to the Salt Cave in Liverpool for being so welcoming and helpful. Without you who knows what kind of state my chest would be in?

To my Dad
Dad, you are someone to look up to no matter how tall I grow.

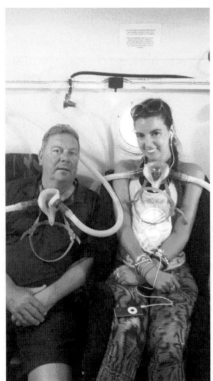

My Dad is the glue that holds my family together; in a time of a crisis he is able to reassure my family and make sure that we support one another. Me and my Dad are like two peas in a pod; throughout this difficult journey he has never once left my side, not just while hospitalised but also at home. He played an important role in my recovery by orchestrating the various tradesmen who were building my own home which was an extension to my family home. To this day, my Dad is still helping me live a normal life. He is the brain behind Mia's Angels, he helps my life run as smoothly as possible by keeping a roof over my head and catering for my every need. When in a meeting, my Dad is my voice, he makes sure that everybody speaks directly to me, without patronising me. If they upset me in any way he is more than willing to show them to the door!

My Dad was a head teacher and had to quit his job that he had worked so hard to get. I am a Daddy's little wild child and always make his hair curl when I do my different adventures. We often still have Daddy-daughter film nights, which are really special to me and he comes to oxygen-therapy session with me too, for moral support. Every morning without fail he would arrive on the hospital ward with his newspaper and flask of coffee, it meant so much and always brightened my day. It makes me cry thinking about it to this day because it shows me the kind of man he is and the devotion he has.

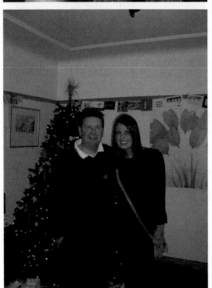

To my Mum
Life doesn't come with a manual, it comes with a mother.

My Mum, also known as Crazy Caz, is the woman that taught me to be strong and I got my kindness from her too. She played another extremely important role while on my journey to recovery. My crazy mother has the ability to lighten any dark moments with joy and laughter. During my time in hospital, my Mum would tease and mess about with me in order to make me feel like my happy self. When I was feeling helpless, my Mum would kidnap me to take me for a spin in my wheelchair around the hospital. I remember one afternoon spelling out to her, 'Mum, what if I try to talk and sound awful?' and she didn't get upset and reassured me, 'As if that would be allowed with your Mum as an English and drama teacher!'.

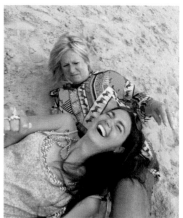

Since I have been left with locked-in syndrome, my Mum has accompanied me on many of my travels. We have visited many countries together, including Morocco and Thailand. Without the company of my Mum, I am one hundred percent certain that my life would not be nearly as happy as it is. We now still do so much together; not only does she come to salt therapy with me, we go shopping together and watch films together. I love spending quality time with her, she keeps things real.

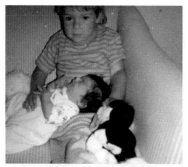

Kelly
20m ago

The Austin siblings 🖤

CHAT

To Sam
Sometimes having a brother is better than having a superhero.

I am the middle child in my family, I have an older brother Sam, and a younger sister Sophie. When growing up, me and my brother were not too close; to be quite honest we didn't like each other much. However, since my accident, he regularly turned up at the hospital and has been there for me whenever I needed him. He is just like my personal body guard, ensuring that nobody could emotionally or physically hurt me and for that, I love him. We have grown to be an exceptionally close-knit family since my accident, mostly because we have been through thick and thin with each other. He is now a respected P.E. teacher and I look up to him. I love the fact that he lives nearby and it's great that we can meet up when we go on nights out sometimes. I do wish we had bonded more before my accident but at that age we were too cool to be associated with each other. But there is no time in life for regrets so we now go out often and make an effort to see each other more.

To Sophie – the other half of me
How do people make it through life without a sister?

But mostly a special thank you to my little sister; you will never understand how incredible you are and your smile lights up my day. Sophie, my younger sister, is my partner in crime, my absolute best friend in the whole world. We are essentially the same person; we love the same thing and we do everything hand in hand (quite literally). As we are so alike, we can have an in-depth conversation in code where no one else knows what we are talking about. Sophie has also accompanied me to many places; we have held monkeys in Morocco and danced in the rain in Thailand. Our promise to each other is to travel the world. I can trust Sophie with every single aspect of my life, from styling my identity to being the keeper of my secrets. Without Sophie, I would not be Mia. She is a mini-me, and she is like my own personal Rottweiler, she takes absolutely no shit. Sophie has three jobs and one includes working for me, which I love because we get sister time. Although I want her to take up her singing, which once woke me up from my coma. We spend loads of time together when we get the chance; we love going on nights out, visiting festivals and on other little adventures to pass the time between our travels. I could write a whole book on how much of an amazing sister she is and I could go on forever about how great she is. She truly is my superhero sister and my soulmate.

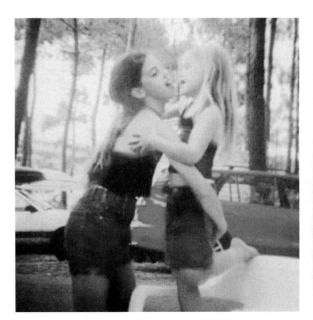 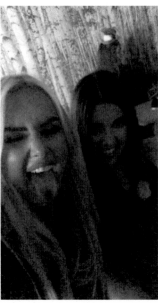

The End

Made in the USA
Coppell, TX
12 March 2020